THE
BODY
BREAKTHROUGH

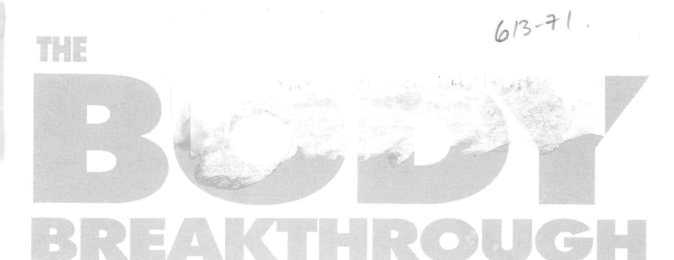

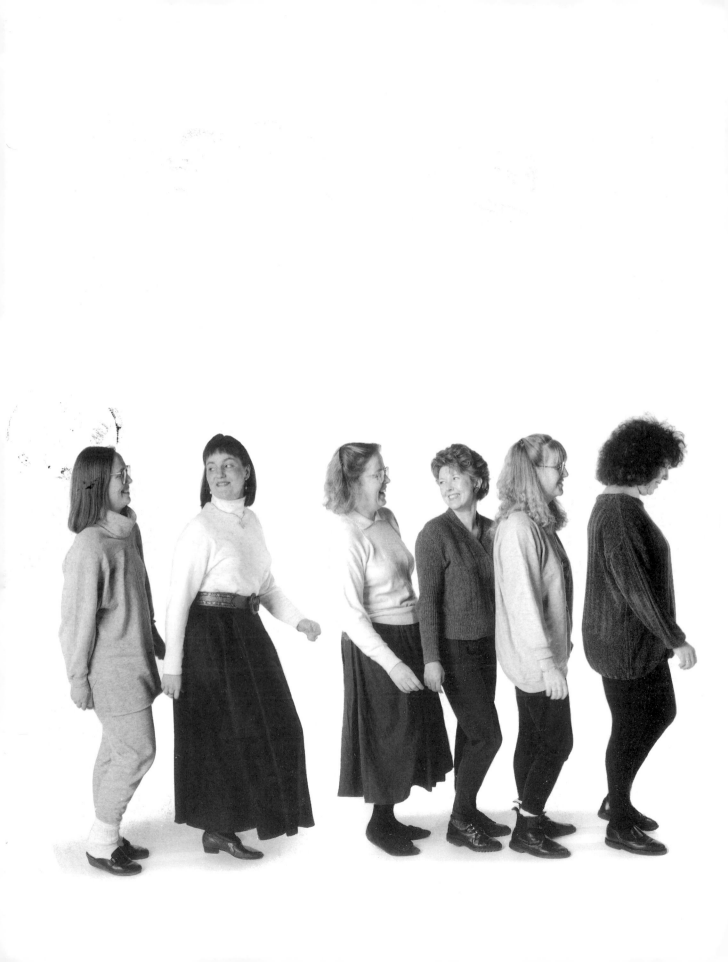

THE
BODY
BREAKTHROUGH

BEL HISLOP

DISCOVER WHICH BODY SHAPE YOU ARE AND UNLOCK THE KEY TO DRAMATIC WEIGHT LOSS

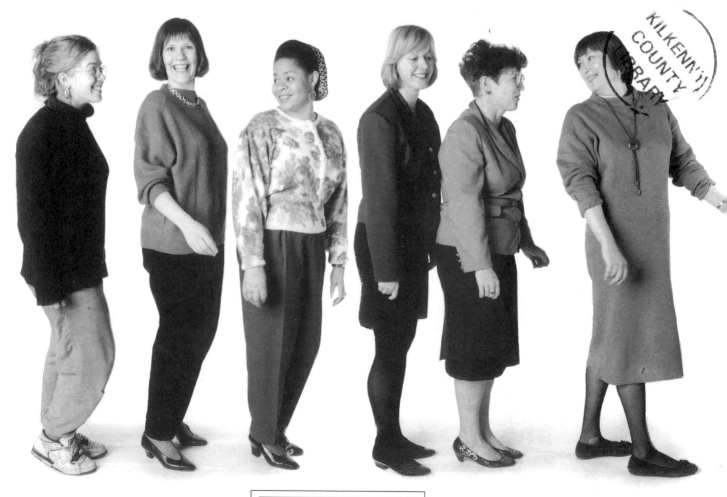

TED SMART

A TED SMART Publication 1995

First published in 1993 by Vermilion
an imprint of Ebury Press
Random House
20 Vauxhall Bridge Road
London SW1V 2SA

Reprinted 1993

A catalogue record for this book is available from the
British Library.

ISBN 0 091 80449 3

Edited by Emma Callery
Designed by Jerry Goldie
Cover photographs by Graham Tann
Photographs by Helen Pask and Jon Stewart
Illustrations by David Downton and Tony Hannaford

Typeset from disk in Goudy by Textype Typesetters,
Cambridge

Printed and bound in Great Britain by
Butler & Tanner Ltd, Frome and London

The author would like to state that the information
contained in this book was checked as rigorously as possible
before going to press. Neither the author nor the publisher
can take responsibility for any changes which may have
occurred since, nor for any other variance of fact from that
recorded here in good faith.

Before beginning the diet and exercise programmes
contained in this book it is advisable to obtain the approval
of your doctor. These programmes are intended for people
of all ages in good health.

The photograph of the Princess of Wales was supplied by
Tim Graham, those of Felicity Kendall and
Princess Stephanie by Rex Features Ltd, and that of
Patricia Hodge by Richard Young for Rex Features Ltd.

For further information on personal and corporate consultations
on image and diet, contact:
WORKING IMAGE, PO Box 3000, London N5 1WW, England

CONTENTS

DISCOVER YOUR

Every woman falls into one of four body-type categories. The type you are can have far-reaching significance in your life; what you eat, how you exercise, what you wear, how you age, what illnesses you are prone to, even how you feel. It is important to be able to identify what body type you are: do you recognise yourself in one of these shapes?

The questionnaire over the page will either reinforce your decision or help you discover exactly which body-type category you fall into.

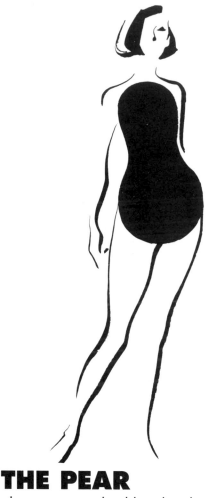

THE PEAR
- has narrower shoulders than hips
- has less fat above the waist than below
- always has a waist and flattish tummy
- has curvy hips and thighs.

THE HOURGLASS
- has balanced shoulders and hips
- has fat equally distributed on bust and hips
- retains a waist however heavy she gets
- always has a curve to her hips however thin she gets.

BODY TYPE

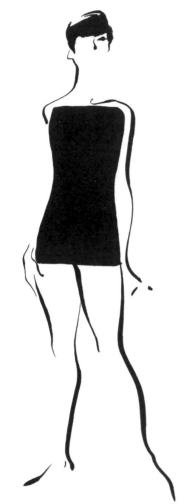

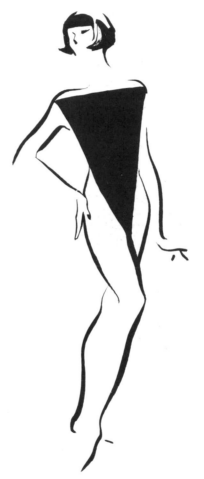

THE RECTANGLE
- has balanced shoulders and hips
- has not got a sharply defined waist
- has a strong body often with slim legs
- has straight hips and a flattish bottom.

THE TRIANGLE
- has broader shoulders than hips
- has a waist and *straight* hips tapering to thighs
- has a narrow pelvis and flat bottom
- has lean lower legs.

QUESTIONNAIRE

For each question, please read alternatives carefully and tick one answer in the boxes at the right hand side

BODY SHAPE

1 **Please look at yourself in a mirror, without your clothes, and face-on. Do you have a body shape with:**
   a shoulder and hip of similar width, with little or no waist?   [C]
   b shoulder and hip of similar width, with a defined waist?   [B]
   c shoulders narrower than hips, with a slim waist?   [A]
   d broader shoulders with tapering hips and a defined waist?   [D]

2a **Now look at yourself sideways. Is your bottom:**
   a flat and tucked in?   [C&D]
   b a more rounded curve?   [A&B]

2b **Still looking sideways, do you carry most weight:**
   a in front of you on bust, tummy and spare tyre (roll of fat above waist)?   [C&D]
   b behind you, on bottom?   [A]
   c equally front and back, on bust and bottom?   [B]

3 **Now looking at yourself from the back, do you have noticeable 'saddlebags' (curvy deposits of fat on the outer thighs)?**
   a No   [C&D]
   b Yes   [A&B]

4 **With a tape measure, measure your waist and then the *biggest* part of your hips. Is your hip measurement:**
   a MORE than 25 cms (10 ins) bigger than your waist?   [A&B]
   b LESS than 25 cms (10 ins) bigger than your waist?   [C&D]

WEIGHT DISTRIBUTION

5 Still looking at yourself in the mirror, face-on and then side-on. When you put on weight is it more noticeable:

a in your face-on body profile, *ie* you get *wider*? [A&B]

b in your side-on body profile, *ie* you get *deeper*? [C&D]

6a When you are/were very slim and put on those *first* 3 kg (7 lbs) of weight, where was it most noticeable:

a *lower* hips and thighs, and a bit on tummy? [B]

b tummy and spare tyre? [C]

c *lower* hips and thighs? [A]

d tummy, upper chest and face? [D]

6b When you are more than 3 kg (7 lbs) overweight, where does your excess weight accumulate:

a on tummy, upper chest, upper arms, *upper* hips, *ie* just below waist, and inside thighs, BUT retaining a waist? [D]

b most on *lower* hips and thighs, little on top half of body? [A]

c pretty much all over, ie on bust and predominantly on hips, BUT retaining a waist? [B]

d on tummy, spare tyre, bust, back and *upper* hips, losing what little waist you might have had? [C]

7 If you were to put on 3 kg (7 lbs) would you get noticeably fatter in the face?

a Yes [C&D]

b No [A&B]

8 If you were to put on 3 kg (7 lbs) would your hands and feet get noticeably more fleshy?

a Yes [B&C]

b No [A&D]

ENERGY LEVELS AND EATING PATTERNS

9 Regardless of demands of work, children, etc, when naturally are you most *mentally* energetic?

a slow to get going, most *creative* energy at night [C]

b physical energy levels pretty constant all day, *creative* energy increases from afternoon into evening [A]

c brightest in the morning, early to bed [D]

d spurts and slumps of *creative* energy throughout the day [B]

10 Regardless of the social and work demands in your life (and when you're not on a diet), which best describes your natural eating habits:

a like to snack through the day [B]

b irregular or erratic meal times, no heavy meals at night [D]

c healthy appetite—start eating can't stop [C]

d can go for quite a long time without food, seldom binge [A]

EXERCISE

11 How sporty were you as a schoolgirl?

a keen to get out of the gym periods and ferocious hockey matches – not at all competitive but happy to play tennis and rounders [A]

b very sporty and enthusiastic, loved athletics, team sports, etc, likely to enter for as many events as possible on Sports Day [C]

c sporty and very competitive, not so keen on team sports but good at individual athletic events, competitive tennis/squash/gymnastics and dancing [D]

d pretty easy-going either way, good at team sports, not very competitive, more interested in the camaraderie [B]

12 **If you want to lose weight, do you:**

a go on a diet and not worry about increasing your exercise? ✓ [A]

b go on a diet and *think* about doing more exercise but not be very enthusiastic about it? [B]

c go on a diet and work out a practical plan for doing more regular exercise—and intend to keep to it? [C]

d you're already doing quite a bit of exercise, so you go on a diet and increase your exercise even more? [D]

13 When you're engaged in a vigorous programme of exercise and sport would you get depressed and put on weight if you gave it up?

a Yes [C&D]

b No ✓ [A&B]

Now add up all the capital letters in the boxes you have ticked.

A predominance of As and you're a **PEAR** type

A predominance of Bs and you're an **HOURGLASS** type

A predominance of Cs and you're a **RECTANGLE** type

A predominance of Ds and you're a **TRIANGLE** type

If you have no clear predominance of any one letter, then add up just the ticks from the *Body Shape* and *Weight Distribution* sections. They are more accurately indicative of your body type.

Finally, check your own physical characteristics against the checklist over the page which will help to clarify your type (but obviously not everyone will conform to *all* the characteristics of their type). The four body types, however, apply to all women, whatever their race or nationality.

If you have passed the menopause and your shape has thickened, particularly around the waist—a Triangle type, for example, can become more like a Rectangle—then answer the questions as if for your original shape and follow the appropriate body-type programme.

THE FOUR BODY TYPES

These illustrations show you exactly where each body type is most likely to put on weight.

THE PEAR

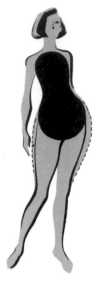

has narrower shoulders than hips
has less fat above the waist than below
always has a waist and flattish tummy
has curvy hips and thighs

If you:

- put weight predominantly on your *lower* hips, bottom and thighs
- have a small bust in proportion to your hips
- have delicate shoulders and neck
- rarely put weight on your shoulders and face

then you are a Pear Type

For your complete four-week diet and exercise package: turn to page 25

THE HOURGLASS

has balanced shoulders and hips
has fat equally distributed on bust and hips
retains a waist, however heavy she gets
always has a curve to her hips however thin she gets

If you:

- put weight on all over, but particularly on *lower* hips and bottom
- have a rounded bosom and rounded bottom
- always keep your waist
- have basically *rounded* limbs

then you are an Hourglass Type

For your complete four-week diet and exercise package: turn to page 49

THE RECTANGLE

has balanced shoulders and hips

has *not* got a sharply defined waist, even when slim

has a strong and sturdy body often with slim legs

has straight hips and a flattish bottom

If you:

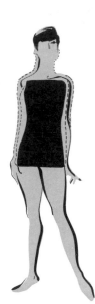

- have lean legs and a flattish bottom which gets fatter and squarer from the waist down
- put weight on torso, predominantly on stomach, spare tyre, breasts, upper back and upper hips
- lose what little waist you have when overweight (become more of a 'cube' than a Rectangle)
- become *deeper*, ie put weight on the front
- have basically *straight* limbs

then you are a Rectangle Type

For your complete four-week diet and exercise package: turn to page 25 *in the reverse section of the book*

THE TRIANGLE

has broader shoulders than hips

has a waist and *straight* hips which taper towards thighs

has a narrow pelvis and a flat bottom

has lean lower legs

If you:

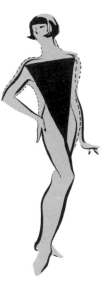

- look top heavy when you put on weight
- put weight on predominantly above the hip bone; on tummy, chest, face, spare tyre, upper arms, *upper* hips and *inner* thighs
- have straight hips which get boxy when overweight
- get fleshy and squarer in the back and chest when overweight

then you are a Triangle Type

For your complete four-week diet and exercise package: turn to page 49 *in the reverse section of the book*

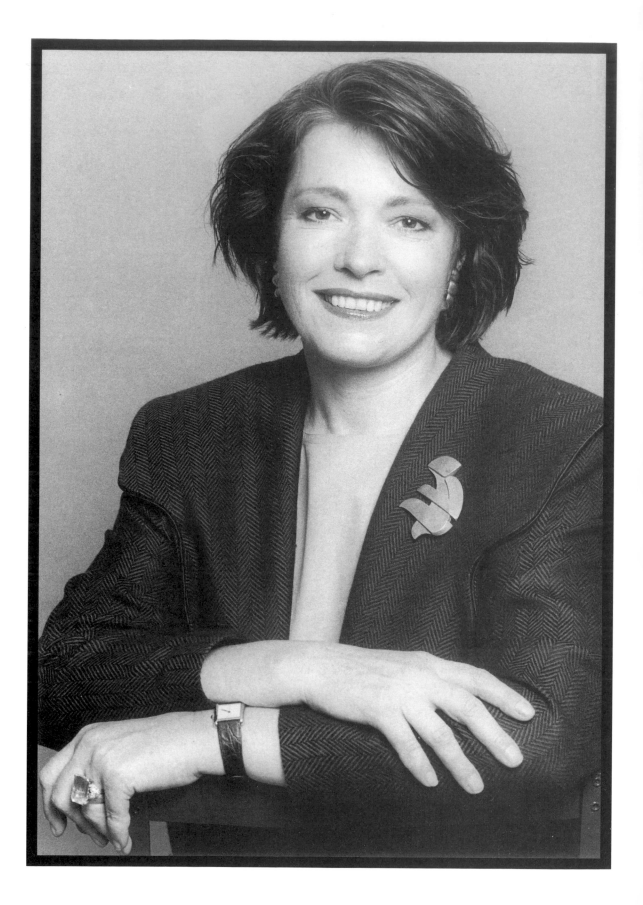

INTRODUCTION

I AM a style and personal development consultant and after years of work and discussion with thousands of women clients and reading of scientific papers, I have discovered a simple truth about women's body shapes—we are not all the same physical type and do not share the same basic shape. Furthermore, our different body shapes indicate different metabolisms and different dietary and exercise needs.

I have always known that I was a different basic shape from my two sisters because what I wore didn't necessarily suit them and vice versa. We also put weight on in different areas and in different proportions. We cannot change this basic underlying shape although we can refine features of it through diet and exercise. But only when I began my training as a style consultant did I realize how important and unchanging these different body shapes are. Which body type you are is significant in many ways, most noticeably in the way your body responds to food and exercise.

This simple fact, that we have different shapes and therefore different metabolisms, is the basis of this book—a breakthrough among diet books. It is backed up by some really remarkable scientific evidence (see below) which has shown that the differences in female body shape and where fat is deposited indicate something of central importance to everyone wishing to understand themselves and their bodies.

This central idea seems to explain an important reason why many women fail in their attempts to become slimmer and fitter, why so many feel deprived or—worse still—ill and debilitated on a diet they may have chosen. Just as there is no one perfect shape for everyone, there is no one diet for everyone.

Bel has been a consultant in personal development for six years with CMB, running her own consultancy in London. Her work has involved her in all aspects of personal presentation and appearance, including the analysis of individual body shapes, colouring and style.

She was aware of the need to help people to make the most of, and to come to terms with, their own individual body shape, and not aspire to unattainable ideals. It has particularly concerned her that most women she worked with were unhappy with some aspect of their bodies and most had been, or were on, a diet—the majority of them ultimately failing.

This book is the result of years of work and thought—and its message is, *we are not all the same*. Find *your* body shape and individual style, dietary and exercise needs—and your personal revolution has begun.

The Scientific Research

The scientific findings as to the significance of female body type are truly revolutionary. One of the early scientific papers which alerted other researchers to the correlation between body shape and metabolism was published in 1983 in the *Journal of Clinical Investigations* by researchers at the University of Gothenburg, Sweden. They divided 670 women into two basic body types; those who put weight on predominantly above the hips (this type of fat distribution follows the male pattern and so this type was called 'android') and those who put on weight predominantly on the lower hips, bottom and thighs (this is the traditional female pear shape, and so was called 'gynoid').

The researchers found that women with upper body adiposity had a predominance of large fat cells which reacted differently from the smaller fat cells characteristic of women with lower body adiposity. But most remarkably they found a significant increase in metabolic aberrations leading to diabetes and heart disease among the top-heavy android type compared with the bottom-heavy gynoid type.

In this Gothenburg paper's own words: 'The present study reports on extensive metabolic and morphologic investigations in 930 obese men and women. The data clearly showed that the men as a group were more susceptible than women to the metabolic aberrations induced by moderate obesity. *However, women with a typical male abdominal type of obesity, also had a metabolic risk profile resembling that of men.* When taken together, the results stressed the importance of the regional distribution of the adipose tissue to the metabolic aberrations that are seen in the obese state.'

The researchers believed that the most likely regulator of whether a

'The principle is absolutely perfect. I felt really good. I wanted to lose 3–4.5 kg (7–10 lbs) and lost 4 kg (9 lbs) easily and quickly but what really amazed me is the loss in inches. Perhaps it's the combination of the foods. It was really important for me to realize how important exercise was. I now do a lot more on a regular basis. I have completely changed my exercise and eating habits.'

Nita
A TRIANGLE TYPE

women is an 'android'- or a 'gynoid' type is the sex-hormones. So it would seem that a gynoid-shaped woman's metabolism is more influenced by female hormones than the top-heavy android body shape, with male-type fat distribution. (And this might explain why, with the volunteer dieters, the Pear and Hourglass type women put on weight more readily from puberty onwards, although the Rectangle-type women caught up with them from their thirties onwards.)

A well-regarded paper published in 1982 from researchers at the Medical College of Wisconsin suggests that 'sites of fat distribution [in women] provide a diagnostic tool to predict abnor- malities in glucose and lipid metabolism.' Most of these researchers use the ratio between waist mea- surement and hip measurement to determine whether a woman patient has a propensity of upper-body fat or lower-body fat (the closer the measurements are, the more 'apple-shaped' and therefore the more upper body fat: whereas a classic 'pear shape' will have a waist measurement significantly smaller than her hip measurement, an indication of lower-body fat).

'I feel really healthy and I've never eaten so much raw food and vegetables. Great. I am delighted with the whole thing.'

Jan
A PEAR TYPE

An interesting follow-up to the Gothenburg paper in 1984 suggests that women with increased upper-body fat should reduce their weight in order to reduce certain specific risks to their health. But it was recommended that further research was necessary to check the extent of this casual relationship: 'Our findings suggest that studies of reduction of body weight and concomitantly of the ratio of waist to hip circumference in subjects in whom this index is increased are urgently needed. The effect of such intervention should be studied with respect to risks for cardiovascular disease.'

An extensive paper published in 1988, 'A Weight Shape Index for Assessing Risk of Disease in 44,820 Women', extended the findings of the previous researchers. This study involved the researchers at the Med- ical College of Wisconsin again but this time with the collaboration of women on a sensible slimming programme with an American non-profit making slimming club. The women were divided into two age groups; 19,947 women in the 20–35 years group were investigated for correlation between body fat distribution and menstrual abnormalities, and 24,873 women in the 40–59 years group were investigated for the prevalence of chronic diseases, diabetes, gall bladder and heart. The paper claimed: 'Upper-body fat predominance results in an increased risk of diabetes, hypertension, gallbladder disease and menstrual abnormalities.'

Dr Mary Loveday, Harley Street allergist and clinical ecologist, also recognises in her diagnostic work the significance of body shape. 'It is so necessary to realise that there is no ideal shape, and that we are born with a certain body type which is our lot. However, what we do (diet and exercise) can enhance that basic shape. I'm so sure that if we are unhappy with the quest for the "ideal" shape then that is the start of anorexia and bulimia.

'I too was intrigued by, and can verify that, the Triangle needs almost masculine exercise –whereas the Pears and Hourglasses hate it and need rather to do the gentle yoga.' Dr Loveday gave a warning that if a woman's basic body shape changes radically then medical opinion ought to be sought. For instance, a woman's thyroid can become over or under active, particularly at menopause, and can change a woman's natural pattern of weight distribution (when, for example, a natural Hourglass might lose her waist).

All women belong to one of four body shapes

Armed with these well-documented scientific facts, I was interested to see how they corresponded with my own findings about women and body shape. As a consultant on dressing and style, I had long recognized the two distinct female types described by the scientists. However, female body shape more accurately sub-divides again to make four classic types. Whether overweight or slim, young or old, any woman can be assigned to one of four body types: the 'Pear' and 'Hourglass' belong to the *gynoid* group and the 'Rectangle' and 'Triangle' belong to the *android* group. To further research the differences between these body types, I sent out 200 extensive questionnaires and the information from them has informed and reinforced the details of the four eating and exercise packages found in this book. One of the significant differences between body types, which backs up the Swedish research of 1983 is that 100 per cent of the Pear-type women responding to the questionnaire said they put on weight, while less than 50 per cent of the Triangle type did (and they were seldom more than 3 kg [7 lbs] heavier than the weight they liked to be). Dr Loveday has also noticed this, pointing out that the gynoid shapes, the Pear and Hourglass, tend to put on more weight during pregnancy then the Rectangle- and Triangle-type women.

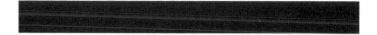

•Felt fitter after starting the diet. Once I started exercising at night I felt *even* fitter. The amount of food allowed per day is ideal.

Brilliant. Easy. I recommend it. . . •

Lindsay
AN HOURGLASS TYPE

Also with the aid of the questionnaire, I began to see that women with different body shapes appeared to have different attitudes towards dieting and exercise. One woman would say that dieting was not enough, she always had to exercise hard if she wanted a significant weight loss; another would insist that just cutting down on her food did all that was necessary and the most exercise she ever needed was a country walk or a bit of yoga, and that hard workouts in the gym were anathema.

Jenny Agutter, a famous 'gynoid' who swears by yoga, is one of these latter women: 'I've always hated aerobics and running, but there's something elegant about yoga.' And, in fact, it is the 'gynoid'-type women, the Pear- and Hourglass-shaped, who were more likely to be getting out of games at school, whereas the 'androids', the Rectangle- and Triangle-shaped women, remained the competitive, sporty types into adulthood. Think of all the leading women tennis players. Maria Bueno was the last gynoid champion and that was decades ago, before really hard-hitting 'masculine' play entered women's tennis.

Jane Fonda, who is on the opposite end of the body shape scale from Jenny Agutter, dedicated the second phase of her career to promoting really tough aerobic exercise for women. Ultimate physical fitness and stamina became a driving necessity for her in a way it never would for a gynoid-type woman. Not only do android-type women crave exercise, the evidence of the scientific papers outlined above would suggest that they actually need to do aerobic exercise to help keep the arterial system healthy as android types are at greater risk of ill health when overweight than are gynoid-shaped women.

There is no one diet to suit everybody

We are bombarded with different diets, but all of them assume we are the same, that we have the same metabolisms and share the same dietary tastes and needs. Most work well for some people, but they do not work for everyone. Some faddy diets can be positively harmful.

In my work, women have expressed distinct differences in their success rate with various diets. The type of food which they ate and the time of eating have been significant factors in the success of a diet. In my experience, body type is also connected to the timing of our peaks of energy. It is better to eat your main meal when your metabolism is most active.

Dieticians have concluded that a diet will be more successful if a woman follows her natural eating and energy pattern. For instance, Rectangle-type women are more awake and active in the evening and therefore feel better and lose weight more efficiently if they have a very light breakfast, a light lunch and then their main meal at night.

That individuals have different dietary needs was made clear to me when I saw two clients, Jane and Christine, within a few days of each other. Both were on the same raw fruit and vegetable diet, but they had

•The diet was so easy to keep to, it actually re-educated my whole attitude to eating, so that I will stick to this system of eating permanently. I gained a lot of energy (as the 39-year-old mother of a two-and-three-quarter year old, a big bonus). I had no difficulty fitting the diet around my family—they adapted to the healthier system—I gave them extra helpings and they had potatoes added if requested. My little daughter and I developed a craving for fresh fruit. My husband loved the chick pea curry.

No calorie-counting was a boon— particularly when eating out. As a vegetarian it was easy to substitute a vegetarian product for the meat dishes.'

Diane
A RECTANGLE TYPE

responded very differently Jane's skin was clearer, she said, than it had been for years: she felt light and full of energy and had lost 3 kg (7 lbs) in two weeks. Christine, on the other hand, was pale and lethargic. She said she felt dreadful and lacked energy and, worse still, did not seem to be losing weight significantly.

I knew that Jane and Christine were different body shapes (a Pear and Triangle respectively) and suggested Christine might try a diet with more protein. Her energy and well-being returned within two days and she started to lose weight.

There is no one ideal shape for everyone

It is sad but true that most women are dissatisfied with at least one part of their bodies and wish they could change it. We have images of 'perfect' female body shapes paraded before us from every medium: we grow up thinking there is one perfect type and most of us are convinced that if only we were not so greedy or lazy we could approximate to this ideal paraded in front of us by the fashion industry and Hollywood. The whole idea of an 'ideal' is made all the more impossible and ridiculous by the fact that it changes with the decades.

'This Pear diet and exercise programme is completely tuned into how I like to live. It makes absolute sense to me that we have different shapes and different metabolisms. I find this diet no hardship at all to follow and am delighted with how easily I have lost weight (6 kg [13 lbs] in six weeks) and how energetic and well I am looking and feeling. I think the whole body-type idea is fascinating and so obviously true. Thank you Bel.'

Jane
A PEAR TYPE

This is one of the most important messages of this book. I feel very strongly that by coming to terms with our shape, it is possible to make the most of it and *love* the body we have. That doesn't mean that we cannot be slimmer and trimmer and fitter generally, if we choose. But it does mean the end of unreasonable expectations and chronic dissatisfaction.

This realization has truly liberated me from the tyranny of the ideal body. The relief in knowing that no amount of exercise and dieting will produce a marked waist and board-flat tummy for me (a Rectangle type) is tremendous. And it also helps me appreciate the good points about my body-type—slim legs, athletic build, strength and endurance. I know I cannot be the typical model-girl shape (Triangle) or a curvy siren shape like Marilyn Monroe or Joan Collins (Hourglass) but I can make the most of what I am. AND SO CAN YOU.

163 kg (358 lbs) in 6 weeks!

The scientific facts and anecdotal evidence helped me formulate an extensive, in-depth questionnaire on dietary and exercise needs which I sent out to 200 women. The results from this gave me the basis for the four body-type diet and exercise programmes. To refine these further, I asked for volunteer dieters to follow the programme designed for their individual body-type for six weeks (some continued much longer). Their experiences and comments helped make the four body-type programmes in this book tailor-made for <u>you</u>.

The progress of these dieters was fantastic. Thirty women divided into the four basic types lost 163 kg (358 lbs) in six weeks! That's an average of nearly 5.5 kg (12 lbs) per person which delighted them and me. Some only had a few kilos to lose (as you can see in the weight and measurement chart with each body-type package), but there were others who had a long way to go. It was they who particularly touched me by their progress: women who had never managed to lose so much before on *any* diet; women who had lost more than 12.5 kg (2 stone) in those six weeks, and those who were lighter than they had been for 20 years.

All these women's lives and spirits were enhanced by their sense of achievement, their greater energy and their pleasure in their looks. And all of them, now months later, have continued to lose weight or maintain their new weight, all saying they have learned a better way of eating *for them* which will be a healthy plan for life.

We had great fun during the six-week experiment. Only two women dropped out, and both for good personal reasons. Everyone else showed such enthusiasm and success that all the hard work of thinking out and planning these programmes was rewarded many times over. Some personal anecdotes of the volunteer dieters are included in each diet and exercise package. It has been a marvellous experience and I am very grateful indeed to all those women whose experiences, suggestions and—best of all—successes have helped me make this book.

Everything that I've learnt about body shape and its significance in all aspects of life, particularly on diet and exercise, is here in this book. My own experience, the experiences of my family, friends and clients, and the scientific papers have all contributed. Now that you've done the questionnaire and discovered your own body type you have the key to your own transformation. Today is the first day of the rest of your life–join us and start now.

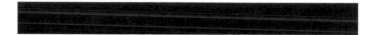

•When I read your introduction to the Hourglass body type I really felt that you were speaking to me personally, almost that you could see into my mind. It was so me.

I didn't feel like I was on a diet. The cottage cheese and fruit for lunch suited me greatly and I've gladly had it every day for eight weeks. Also the chick pea curry was delicious.

I've bought a new leotard to replace my usual baggy top.⁹

Denise
AN HOURGLASS TYPE

References

Kissebah, Ahmed H. et al., 1982: Relation of Body Fat Distribution to Metabolic Complications of Obesity. *Journal of Clinical Endocrinology and Metabolism.* Vol. 54, No.2, pp. 254–259.

Krotkiewski, Marcin et al., 1983: Impact of Obesity on Metabolism in Men & Women: Importance of Regional Adipose Tissue Distribution. *Journal of Clinical Investigations.* Vol. 72, September 1983, pp. 1150–1162.

Lapidus, Leif et al., 1984: Distribution of Adipose Tissue and Risk of Cardiovascular Disease and Death: a 12 year follow up of participants in the population study of women in Gothenburg, Sweden. *British Medical Journal.* Vol. 289, 10th November 1984, pp. 1257–1261.

Alfred A. Rimm, Arthur J. Hartz and Mary E. Fischer, 1988: A Weight Shape Index for Assessing Risk of Disease in 44,820 Women. *Journal of Clinical Epidemiology.* Vol. 41, No. 5, pp. 459–465, 1988.

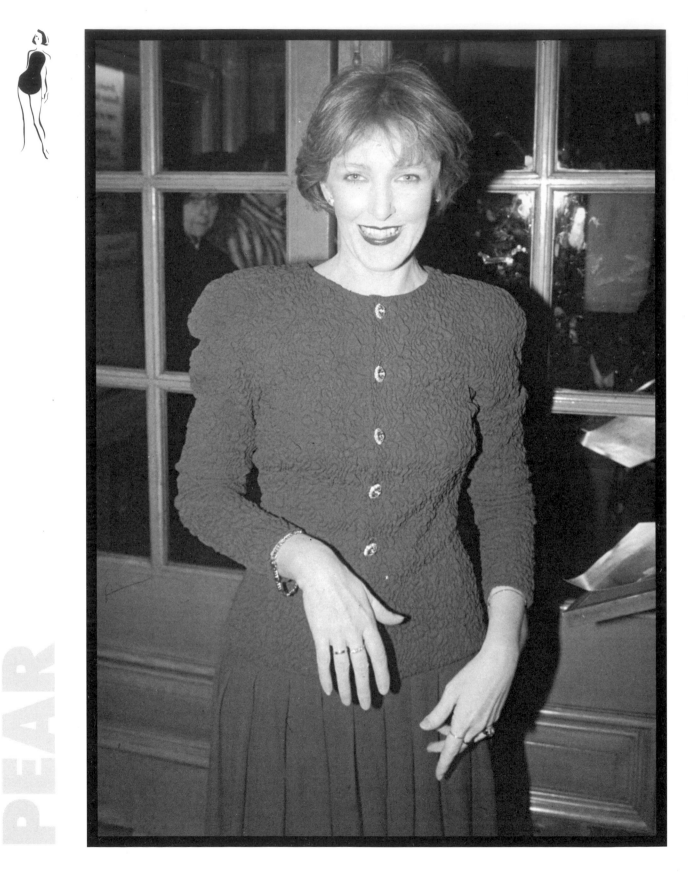

PEAR

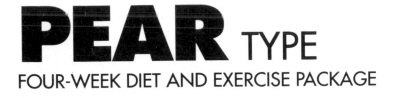

PEAR TYPE

FOUR-WEEK DIET AND EXERCISE PACKAGE

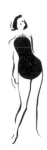

THIS IS a four-week package of diet menus and exercise programmes tailor-made for your body type and metabolism. A team of volunteer dieters tested this diet and exercise programme for six weeks, and some for three months and more. Their experiences and comments went into improving it for you. With each week, my volunteer dieters and I found it was very encouraging to have a treat, or 'positive action', to keep our spirits up and keep us going for the next week. As you read through the package you will see what I mean.

Individual characteristics

The Pear type has a steady energy which tends to be at its lowest in the morning and peak in the evening. Strenuous exercise does not appeal to her, although exercises such as yoga and relaxed swimming which enhance suppleness and grace do.

If she has a basically sedentary job, does no formal exercise and is content with her life, her metabolism can become rather sluggish. Introduce some emotional drama, however—whether falling in love, being suddenly catapulted into the limelight at work, or having to deal with unpleasant office politics—and this type's metabolism can be so energized with excitement or anxiety that she can lose 3 kg (7 lbs) in a week. Doing more exercise, such as walking, swimming, floor exercises, also keeps this type of metabolism burning.

The Pear type will lose weight best and feel most happy and energetic (and therefore more likely to stick to the regime) if she eats plenty of low-fat dairy foods such as cottage cheese and yogurt, and fruit and raw vegetables galore.

Patricia Hodge is an elegant Pear type who has impeccable style. She wears lots of simple, fluid and feminine clothes and is very good at balancing her hippy shape with rounded shoulder pads, as you see with this dress. This soft fabric and gently-fitted bodice shows off her neat upper body and small waist and the softly pleated skirt skims over her broader hips.

Note how delicate her face and hands are: this body type retains her slim face and hands while other body types can thicken in these areas. This dress suits her well; the curvy bodice following the line of her body, the skirt loose over her hips and thighs. Patricia Hodge is particularly successful at dressing to make the most of her feminine shape.

PEAR

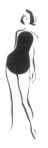

PEAR-TYPE WEIGHT AND MEASUREMENTS BEFORE DIETING, AND SIX WEEKS LATER

| | WEIGHT (kg/st & lbs) | | MEASUREMENTS (cms/ins) | | | | | |
| | | | BEFORE | | | AFTER | | |
NAME	BEFORE	AFTER	BUST	WAIST	HIPS	BUST	WAIST	HIPS
Karen	79/12 7	73.3/11 9	95/38	77.5/31	110/44	92.5/37	72.5/29	102.5/41
Michelle	50.5/8 0	49.5/7 12	81/32½	61/24½	89/35½	81/32½	60/24	86/34½
Jan	64/10 2	56.7/9 0	87.5/35	69/27½	102.5/41	87.5/35	65/26	95/38
Judy	76.5/12 2	72/11 6	97.5/39	75/30	109/43½	91/36½	72.5/29	106/42½
Jane	69.3/11 0	63.5/10 1	92.5/37	70/28	105/42	90/36	67.5/27	97.5/39
Caroline	71/11 4	64/10 2	94/37½	72.5/29	102.5/41	90/36	67.5/27	97.5/39

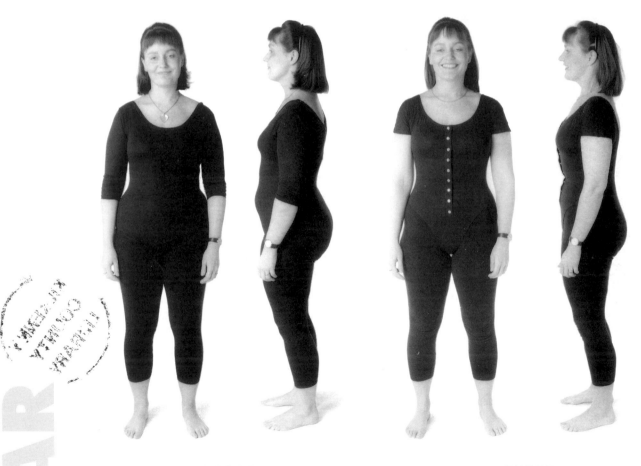

BEFORE

AFTER

Our volunteer above lost 7.2 kg (16 lbs) in weight in the six weeks. She is markedly slimmer from the waist down with again more inches off her waist and hips— 5 cm (2 ins) from each—and 3.75 cm (1½ ins) from her bust. Although Pear types put on weight on their faces last of all, it is good to her see beautiful cheekbones more emphasized and her face generally refined.

PEAR

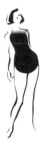

PEAR-TYPE DIETERS' WEIGHT LOSS OVER SIX WEEKS (kg/lbs)

NAME	WEEK:	1	2	3	4	5	6	TOTAL WEIGHT LOSS
Karen		2.7/6	0.5/1	0.5/1	0/0	0/0	+1.8/4	−5.5/12
Michelle		1.8/4	0.5/1	0/0	+0.5/1	+0.5/1	0.5/1	−1.8/4
Jan		2.7/6	1.8/4	0.9/2	0/0	0/0	1.8/4	−7.2/16
Judy		1.8/4	0.9/2	0.5/1	0.5/1	0.5/1	0.5/1	−4.5/10
Jane		1.8/4	0.9/2	0.5/1	0.9/2	0.5/1	1.4/3	−5.9/13
Caroline		3.1/7	0.5/1	0.5/1	0.5/1	0.5/1	2.2/5	−7.2/16

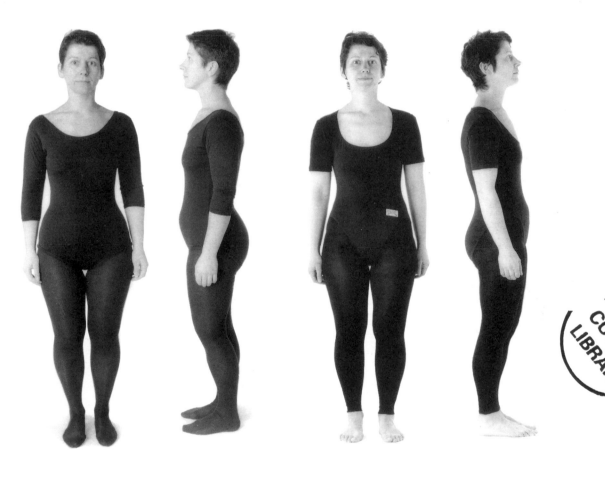

BEFORE

AFTER

Our volunteer above also lost a total of 7.2 kg (16 lbs) in weight in the six weeks – most of it off her hips with a 7.5 cms (3 ins) reduction, 3.75 cms (1½ ins) off her waist and nothing from her bust. Pear-shape women are always smallest on top and put on weight below the waist. This volunteer's weight gain had emphasized her Pear shape, but after her weight loss there is a better sense of balance between her top and bottom halves. Her tummy and bottom are noticeably flatter.

PEAR

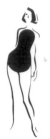

WEEK ONE
Positive action: enhance your style

AS YOU'VE already seen, we don't all share the same body shape and an outfit that looks fantastic on one person can look dreadful on somebody else. And this is not just a matter of slenderness. Wearing clothes which suit your body shape, drawing attention to your good points and hiding your not so good, can give you the appearance of having *lost 3 kg (7 lbs)* before you even begin your diet.

The classic Pear has smaller shoulders and torso than hips. Meryl Streep and Miranda Richardson are two actresses with this body type. Television presenter Anne Diamond is another. Her face rarely puts on weight and her shoulders, back and neck always have a slim, delicate look to them. Whatever your size, you'll always have a waist and this needs emphasizing. The basic principle of style is that you wear clothes which have the same or similar line to your body line. So jackets and tops should be shaped to the waist unless you're very overweight when you may feel happier in something less fitted. But even so, keep that jacket in a soft and draping fabric, like wool crêpe, silk or linen.

Generally speaking, jackets should have soft, rounded shoulder pads, curvy lapels, curved rather than angular hemlines, and be softly fitted to the waist. Fabrics should not be too crisp; keep away from gaberdine, but fine wools, silk, linen and better quality viscoses and rayons are fine. Blouses and tops in delicate, feminine fabrics like fine laces, chiffon, organza and fine cottons all suit the Pear type.

Straight skirts are always a problem for the Pear-shaped woman, even if she is slim. The straightest she should go in a skirt is a tulip-shaped skirt with a couple of soft pleats easing from the waist to the hips. Otherwise a gathered or a riding skirt will be most flattering.

The same is true about trousers. Straight-hipped, masculine-cut jeans or trousers are much too big on the waist and tight across the lower hips and top of thigh. Much more flattering are trousers with a couple of soft pleats from the front waistband easing into loose legs which taper to the ankle. Again, soft, fluid fabrics are best, nothing too stiff or military.

Pear types do have disproportionately delicate shoulders in comparison to their wider hips, and whatever your size some padding at the shoulder, even in blouses, helps balance your body shape. Remember that all details in clothing and accessories should tend towards the curve rather than the straight—collars, lapels, handbags, belt buckles.

If you are very overweight

If this is the case you may feel happier with a slightly modified style. There is a tendency for overweight women to try to camouflage everything and some end up wearing a tent in despair. But all shapes, even carrying a lot of extra weight, still have their distinctive good points and clothes should show these to advantage.

As a Pear type puts on most of her weight below the waist, keep your skirts gently gathered (not too bulky) and in a soft material. The length is important, not too long unless you are tall—experiment in front of a mirror. Keep the emphasis on your waist with a good belt but wear either longer jackets, coming well below your widest point, or shorter jackets, finishing just below the waist. Beware of jackets which end just at your widest hip level and be careful not to wear jackets with shoulders which are too large .

Your top half will be smaller and more delicate than your hips and it is important not to swamp yourself with a jacket in too heavy a style or fabric. You will feel happier in less fitted styles than I have recommended in the general guidelines, going for a straighter style jacket but in a soft fabric like a linen or washed silk, perhaps in a marvellous colour. Don't forget rounded shoulder pads really help this body type, they give a sense of balance to your body and minimize the width of your hips.

Your face and neck are least likely to be heavy and so draw attention to this area of your body with a good coloured blouse or jacket, a lovely scarf, or with a special piece of jewellery, a necklace or brooch to match your style.

Pear types often have small delicate feet and it is a good idea to wear really pretty shoes or ankle

PEAR

boots to draw attention to them. As with all Pear-type accessories, keep details curved: toes almond-shaped, heels delicate, laced-up ankle boots in soft leather or suede, buckles and bows all suit your look.

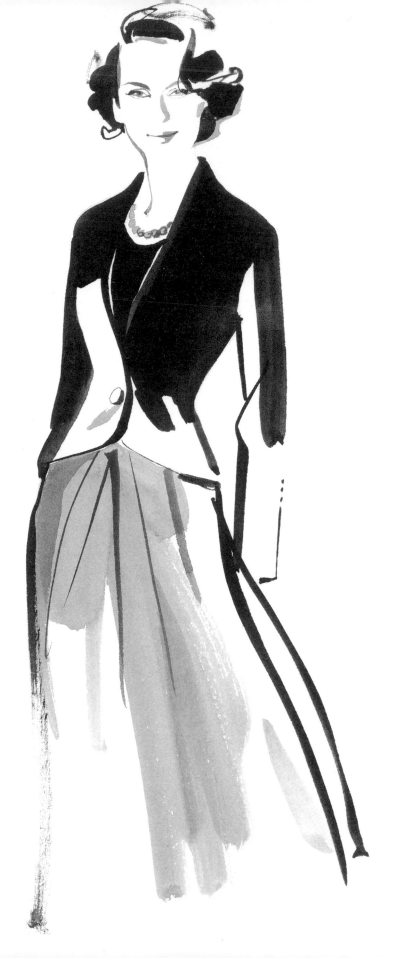

PEAR

29

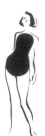

WEEK ONE

Jewellery

Jewellery for the Pear type follows the same line as her body and her clothes. Keep detail curvy: any chain links or beads should be round or oval rather than geometric and flat; curb-link bracelets rather than brick-link for instance. Because you tend to have slim shoulders and neck, necklaces are very pretty on you—and pearls look fabulous on both the curvy shapes, you and the Hourglass.

Similarly, brooches should have swept, curvy lines rather than be too geometric. Organic images—flowers, leaves, wings, crescent moons, serpentine squiggles—all have the necessary curve for this type.

But remember, scale is as important in jewellery as it is in clothes. It has to be the right size for you. If you are large boned (as a rough guide if your wrist measures 16.5cms [6½ins] or more) then your jewellery pieces ought to be large and important. If you are medium (14 to 16.5cms [5½ to 6½ins]) to small boned (less than 14cms [5½ins]) then make sure your jewellery is more delicate and of smaller scale so that it doesn't overwhelm you.

Watches should have round or oval faces and not be too big in the face, or heavy in the bracelet or strap, unless you are big-boned yourself.

So, as your first positive action, make yourself feel better and look slimmer in the right clothes and accessories for your shape. Then, confidence boosted by your new appearance, start on the first week of your own tailor-made diet and exercise plan and begin to lose pounds of real weight.

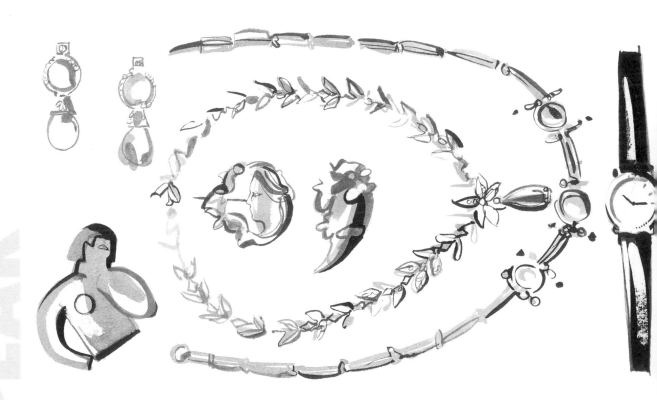

PEAR

30

Starting your diet

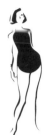

This is a low-fat diet. With a reduced fat, reduced sugar and increased fibre intake, this diet takes into account the latest findings on healthy nutrition. There is a good deal of evidence that this body type particularly thrives on a diet high in raw fruit and vegetables.

The menus which follow are for those of you who like a structured diet. For the rest, they are suggestions for meals based on the basic principles of your body-type diet of low-fat protein (like cottage cheese or white fish), unrefined carbohydrates (like baked potato, wholemeal bread, brown rice), with almost limitless salad and vegetables, and generous amounts of fruit. The Pear type can have her main meal at either lunchtime or in the evening, but she must keep her breakfast very light or even non-existent.

You can switch meals around from day to day—or repeat easy or favourite ones—as long as you have one lunch meal and one supper meal each day. Useful, though not ideal, if you are too busy, or disinclined to cook, are the ready-made, low-calorie frozen meals. You may substitute these for your main meal but add a salad or some vegetables. This diet should not only help the Pear type to lose weight but to be healthier, look better and feel great.

This diet does not allow for alcohol. There are two main reasons for this: alcohol represents empty calories and I would rather you got food value for your extra calories in the shape of an extra piece of fruit, or another helping of salad or vegetables—or even a slightly larger helping of protein: fish or eggs or chicken. But most importantly, alcohol undermines our self-control—and can be addictive. Once we've had one drink it's much easier to have another, and then our resolve goes too and we're eating anything that comes our way.

It's much easier and more efficient if you can cut out alcohol for the duration of your diet. Many women find that they can lose weight just by doing this, so unaware were they of how many extra calories they were consuming every day in liquid form.

However, I am aware that for some women this is an impossibility and if it is the difference between going on the diet or not, obviously I would rather you follow the dieting guidelines and limit your alcohol to one drink a day, preferably with your meal.

DAILY ALLOWANCE
300 ml (½ pt) skimmed milk
15 g (½ oz) low-fat spread

Beverages: try to keep your intake of tea/coffee to two cups a day, but drink plenty of water and have as many cups of herb tea as you like

Unlimited vegetables (preferably raw, otherwise boiled/steamed):

asparagus	aubergine	bean sprouts	beetroot
broccoli	brussel sprouts	cabbage	carrots
cauliflower	celery	chard	chicory
courgettes	cucumbers	French beans	endive
escarole	green/red pepper	kale	lettuce
mange-tout peas	mushrooms	okra	onions
parsley	radishes	runner beans	spinach
spring greens	tomatoes	turnips	watercress

One piece of fruit extra to meal allowances:

apple	apricot	handful blackberries	grapefruit
kiwi	nectarine	orange	peach
pear	plum	tangerine	watermelon, 1 slice

31

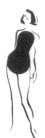

WEEK ONE

For vegetarians there are recipes for main meal substitutions in the recipe supplement on pages 72–9.

DAY ONE
Breakfast
One piece of fruit, cup of tea or coffee, skimmed milk from daily allowance.
Lunch
150 g (5 oz) cottage cheese with one chopped-up apple and orange, piece of wholemeal bread, cup of tea. (Many Pear-type dieters find this the perfect lunch for them, you may choose to have it most days instead of the other suggestions.)
Supper
175 g (6 oz) white fish, grilled or steamed, green salad (as much as you like), low-cal dressing (either commercial brand or home-made [see recipe, page 72]), 150 g (5 oz) low-fat fruit yogurt.

DAY TWO
Breakfast
Same as above.
Lunch
Two hard-boiled eggs chopped into large mixed salad (from permitted vegetables), low-cal dressing (see recipe, page 72), cup of tea.
Supper
Vegetable casserole (see recipe, page 73), wholemeal bread or roll, two-fruit salad and 15 ml (1 tbsp) low-fat natural yogurt.

DAY THREE
Breakfast
Same as above.
Lunch
Baked potato with low-cal coleslaw or homemade with creamy low-cal dressing (see recipe, page 72), 150 g (5 oz) pot low-fat fruit yogurt, cup of tea.

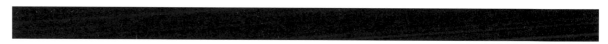

'I am a vegetarian and also allergic to dairy produce so I had to amend my diet from cottage cheese, milk, etc. to fish, eg tuna, salmon, and soya milk and nuts.

I make an effort to increase exercise to two to three runs per week, and a little mountain biking. The exercises specifically for the Pear-shape type were very good. I also now do 10–15 minutes of Callanetic exercises each morning to keep me supple and toned.

An excellently planned diet which can be taken into one's future eating habits for the rest of one's life—not just short term.'

Michele

PEAR

Supper
100 g (4 oz) fresh or tinned salmon, steamed vegetables (from permitted vegetables), fresh fruit salad (from permitted fruit).

DAY FOUR

Breakfast
Same as above.

Lunch
150 g (5 oz) cottage cheese, green salad with olives, radishes and spring onions, low-cal dressing (see recipe, page 72), apple, cup of tea.

Supper
Spaghetti with broccoli (see recipe, page 74), baked pepper salad (see recipe, page 77), slice of wholemeal bread, banana split (1 tbsp iced vanilla yogurt instead of ice cream).

DAY FIVE

Breakfast
Same as above.

Lunch
Pitta bread spread with 50 g (2 oz) hummus, sliced tomatoes, lettuce; 150 g (5 oz) low-fat natural yogurt with one piece of fruit chopped in, cup of tea.

Supper
Quarter chicken roasted, steamed or grilled, big salad or selection of vegetables from permitted list, baked apple with 1 tsp honey and 1 tbsp frozen yogurt.

DAY SIX

Breakfast
Same as above.

Lunch
150 g (5 oz) low-fat natural yogurt, two pieces fruit chopped in, sprinkling of sunflower seeds (optional).

Supper
Salade Niçoise (see recipe, page 76), wholemeal bread, glass unsweetened fruit juice.

DAY SEVEN

Breakfast
Same as above.

Lunch
Baked potato, creamy low-cal dressing (see recipe, page 72), baked pepper and anchovy (see recipe, page 77), one piece of fruit, cup of tea.

Supper 150 g (5 oz) white fish baked, steamed or grilled, two tomatoes and one medium onion, sliced onto lettuce, low-cal dressing (see recipe, page 72), small bunch of grapes.

'So much intelligent thought has gone into this programme. The diet really seems made for me. The style pointers are excellent too and have made such a difference to my self-confidence. I can't believe how much better I am looking, my skin is firmer and clearer than ever —and my clothes really look as if they suit me, instead of someone else! And best of all: the pounds are dropping off and I feel they will stay dropped. I've now got the confidence to turn my energies to other things.'

Caroline

PEAR

33

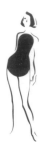

WEEK ONE
Your exercise programme

The Pear type is not one of nature's natural athletes. She does not feel at home in a sweaty gym trying to out-muscle the men, nor is she a highly competitive games-player who pushes herself to the limit on squash or tennis court.

But this body type is supple and graceful and finds that non-aerobic exercise like yoga, Callanetics and relaxed swimming suits her needs particularly well. Luckily, hard exercise is not essential to her fitness or well-being and she can get away with doing much less than can the other types.

Exercise, however, does help everyone to lose weight by burning more calories (half an hour's brisk walking uses up 180 calories) and by boosting the basal metabolic rate for a few hours after the exercise has ceased, continuing to burn more calories. Exercise also helps to tone-up muscles and to increase suppleness and strength.

There is also a 'feel good' factor to exercising which cannot be ignored. If you're doing the exercise that suits your body type and disposition it undoubtedly lifts the spirits, makes you generally more positive about yourself, more in tune with your body—and less likely to neglect and abuse it.

I encourage the Pear type to introduce more formal exercise into her week: swimming twice a week; or walking every day an extra mile to work or shops; or running up stairs rather than taking the lift. I also include three floor exercises, and an additional one in your third week, to be done every day to tone the stomach, hip and thigh muscles.

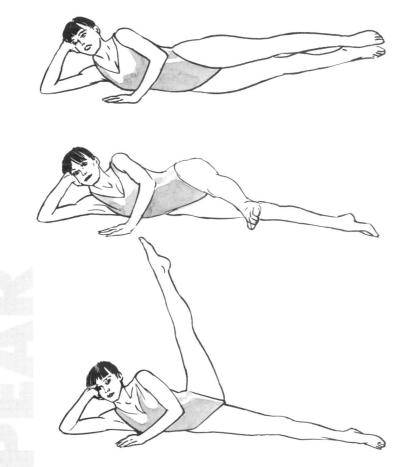

Hip and thigh toner

This will involve the muscles which run from your hips down the outside edge of your thighs. Keep your body in a straight line during the whole exercise.

1 Lie on your right side, supporting your head with your right arm, both legs straight.

2 Slowly raise both legs a few inches off the floor, keeping them as straight as possible. *Hold the position while you count to five.* Then lower.

3 Keeping your body in a straight line raise your left leg into the air until it is at a right angle to your hip.

4 Slowly lower it across your body, keeping your leg straight, and with your foot as close to shoulder level as possible. Hold your extended foot just above ground level *and count to five.*

5 Raise leg again into the air and return to starting position.

6 Raise both legs together off floor as in Step 2. *Hold the position while you count to 30.* Lower legs to floor.

7 Turn over and repeat whole exercise with other leg.

REPEAT EXERCISE TWO TIMES.

PEAR

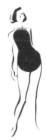

Stomach and waist trimmer

This is an exercise which has a vigorous effect on the muscles of the stomach. You must do it carefully and accurately so that it does not strain your back at all. The moment your back hurts you should stop, this is a sign that you are not using your stomach muscles properly. Follow the instructions carefully.

1 Lie flat on your back on a carpet or folded blanket, with your knees bent and your feet tucked under a bed or sofa, and hands by your sides.

2 Tighten your buttock muscles, round your shoulders and stretch your arms forwards. Making sure your lower back is *pressed* into the floor, slowly pull yourself up using your tummy muscles until your body is quarter-sitting, curled forwards towards your knees and looking a little like a cradle. *Keep the small of your back on the floor all the time.*

3 Thinking of your tummy muscles as strong bands of elastic, reach forward and then move slightly back. *Repeat the whole gentle movement to and fro three times.*

4 Uncurl your spine and slowly lower your upper back and shoulders to the floor. Press small of back into the carpet.

REPEAT EXERCISE THREE TIMES.

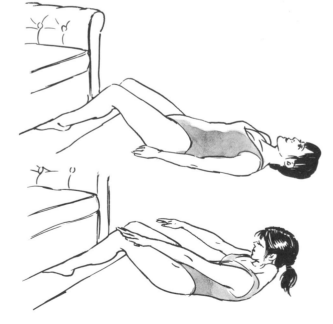

Whole leg toner

Keep your spine straight while doing this exercise (there is a tendency to lean backwards). It will make the tops of your thighs ache, but you know that means unaccustomed muscles are being toned-up and strengthened.

1 Stand sideways beside a chair or chest. Rest hand lightly on the top.

2 Slightly bend the knee which is closest to the chest or chair and keep it in this position throughout the exercise.

3 Slowly lift your other leg up straight in front of you, toes pointed, as high as you can go *and hold the position while you count to five.*

4 Slowly lower your leg. Repeat twice more.

5 Turn round and repeat the movement with the other leg.

REPEAT WHOLE EXERCISE TWO TIMES.

PEAR

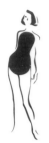

WEEK TWO
Positive action: instant healthy glow

GO AND buy yourself a blusher. Nothing lifts the contours of a face and the colour of a complexion more immediately and naturally than blusher. Buy a powder in a neutral rosy tone and apply it as shown in the illustration below.

1 Brush blush along the cheekbone, starting on a level with the outer edge of your iris and feathering it upwards and outwards as far as the hairline at the top of your ear.

2 You might like also to add the slightest touch of colour to your temples and chin.

3 Blend the edges with a soft powder brush. Never have definite lines in any make-up you apply.

Many women say to me that they don't use make-up and it usually means they are not confident about using it and don't like a made-up look. My answer is that from our mid-twenties onwards our colouring tends to fade and the definition of our features softens with age. I never advocate a stagey effect, but do point out that if you are in business, well-applied make-up gives your features greater definition and adds more authority to your whole image.

If you still feel reluctant or lacking in competence, try using just your new blusher and a soft neutral lipstick and see if you like the effect. This should make your complexion brighter, your eyes more intense in colour and your face more contoured.

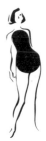

Subtly applied eye make-up needs a bit more technique and practice. But it is eye make-up which most fair-skinned, light-eyelashed women particularly feel they need. In my classes, even the most tentative women manage a professional job after experimenting for half an hour. Without being able to advise you personally, taking into account your individual colouring and shape of eye, I can only give the following steps as a general pointer.

Although Pear types put on weight on their faces last of all, you may well be noticing that your first week's dieting has begun to reveal more marked cheekbones and a cleaner jawline. Certainly, on this diet your skin will improve, although you may find that during the first week it's a bit spotty as you clear some of the toxins out of your system.

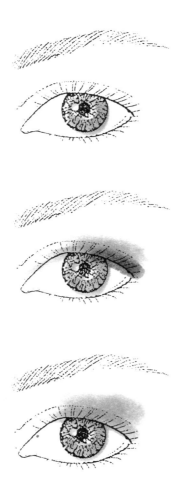

1 Highlighter: using an eyeshadow sponge, apply a light, neutral colour on the whole area of your upper eye from eyelid to brow.

2 Lid: apply a light to medium colour just on the lid (a taupe or soft olive suit most people), blending with a small brush.

3 Orbital bone: apply a darker colour along the upper eye-socket crease, blending it onto the lid at the outer corner of the eye. Blend all the colours with a soft brush. The end result must look like a wash of colour over your lid, getting darker towards the socket and the outside edge. No stripes or hard edges please.

4 Mascara: finish the look off with a couple of coats of brown mascara on the upper lashes, and one coat on the lower.

PEAR

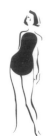

WEEK TWO
Your diet

DAY EIGHT

Breakfast
One piece of fruit, cup of tea or coffee, skimmed milk from your daily allowance.

Lunch
Two-egg omelette with mixed herbs, green beans and carrots, or any two vegetables from the permitted list, 150 g (5 oz) low-fat fruit yogurt, cup of tea.

Supper
100 g (4 oz) peeled prawns, large mixed salad, creamy low-cal dressing (see recipe, page 72), wholemeal bread, two-fruit salad, 1 tbsp frozen yogurt.

DAY NINE

Breakfast
Same as above.

Lunch
100 g (4 oz) cottage cheese with apple and orange chopped in, wholemeal bread, cup of tea.

Supper
Ratatouille (see recipe, page 74), 50 g (2 oz) brown rice, green salad, low-cal dressing (see recipe, page 72), piece of fruit.

DAY TEN

Breakfast
Same as above.

Lunch
Baked potato, 1 tbsp hummus, mixed salad, low-cal dressing (see recipe, page 72), 150 g (5 oz) low-fat fruit yogurt, cup of tea.

Supper
175 g (6 oz) chicken breast, rubbed with 1 tsp olive oil and herbs, grilled, selection of vegetables from permitted list, baked apple with 1 tsp honey and 1 tbsp low-fat natural yogurt.

DAY ELEVEN

Breakfast
Same as above.

Lunch
300 ml (½ pt) any non-creamy packet soup or homemade vegetable soup (see recipe, page 75), one piece wholemeal bread/toast, banana, cup of tea.

Supper
Mushroom omelette (see recipe, page 76), large mixed salad, low-cal dressing (see recipe, page 72), two-fruit salad.

DAY TWELVE

Breakfast
Same as above.

Lunch
100 g (4 oz) cottage cheese, baked pepper salad (see recipe, page 77), one piece of fruit, cup of tea.

Supper
Seafood pasta (see recipe, page 74), green salad, low-cal dressing (see recipe, page 72), one piece of fruit.

DAY THIRTEEN

Breakfast
Same as above.

Lunch
Tabbouleh (see recipe, page 77) in wholemeal pitta bread, cup of tea.

Supper
150 g (5 oz) smoked haddock, steamed or poached in skimmed milk and water, two or more vegetables from permitted list, one piece of fruit cut up into 150 g (5 oz) low-fat natural yogurt.

DAY FOURTEEN

Breakfast
Same as above.

Lunch
Three fruits from permitted list made into fruit salad with 100 g (4 oz) low-fat natural yogurt, cup of tea.

Supper
Quarter of chicken, grilled or dry roasted, large mixed salad, low-cal dressing (see recipe, page 72), wholemeal roll, one piece of fruit.

Your exercise programme

Increase the number of times you repeat the floor exercises described in Week One by one. You should be feeling fitter by now in your daily life, feel more like running up the stairs at work for instance, or perhaps beginning to swim regularly now that you're seeing some of the good effects of your first week's dieting and exercise regime.

You may feel like borrowing an exercise video, like Callanetics or yoga, or some other low- to medium-impact aerobics. It works best if you can make a regular date once or twice a week and exercise with a friend. Or better still, join an exercise class.

EXERCISE REPETITIONS: WEEK TWO	
Whole Leg Toner	3
Hip and Thigh Toner	3
Stomach and Waist Trimmer	4

●I've never been so happy on a diet. It seems to suit me perfectly—the eating routine and the sorts of food suggested could have been tailor-made for me.

I'm lighter now than I have been for 20 years so this is the first diet that has managed to shift the ancient fat. It is also the first diet that I have managed to stick with. The way it's worked for me is that I've dieted quite strictly for a month or six weeks, losing about 3–4.5 kg (7–10 lbs) and then I've eased off for a bit, but still following the basic eating routine of light breakfast, light lunch and main meal in the evening, and during the less strict stages I have managed not to put on any weight. Then after two, three or even sometimes four weeks, I've felt ready to go back on the diet to knock off the next 3 kg (7 lbs). And this has worked for me.

I'm thrilled with my weight loss and feel very grateful to you for introducing me to this whole new way of tackling my problem.●

Karen

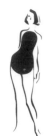

WEEK THREE
Positive action: good foundations

YOU ARE due for a reward for having got this far and lost those first pounds—some of you may be as much as 3 kg (7 lbs) lighter by this point, others more like 1.8–2.3 kg (4–5 lbs). Whatever weight you have lost, you will notice a flattening of the bulges and you may well feel like treating yourself to an indulgence that does not involve food. I suggest a glamorous piece of underwear which will make you feel pampered and proud of your curvy body.

Women with straight hips are more flattered by sporty underwear, but you—a woman with curvy hips and a waist—can get away with frilly, lacy underwear. A pretty underwired, low-cut lace bra will make the most of your small breasts and good shoulders. You are the type of woman who may find it fun to wear the legendary Wonderbra (which some party-goers are wearing as outer wear), which is lacy, low-cut, uplifted and padded for extra curve. Or you may prefer to buy yourself a pair of knickers. Your body type can wear frilly French knickers or lace-trimmed bikinis. Spoil yourself!

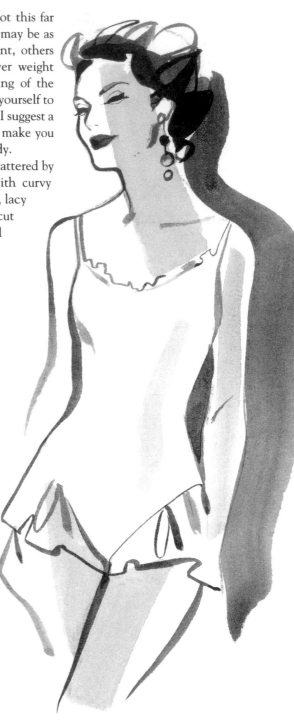

PEAR

40

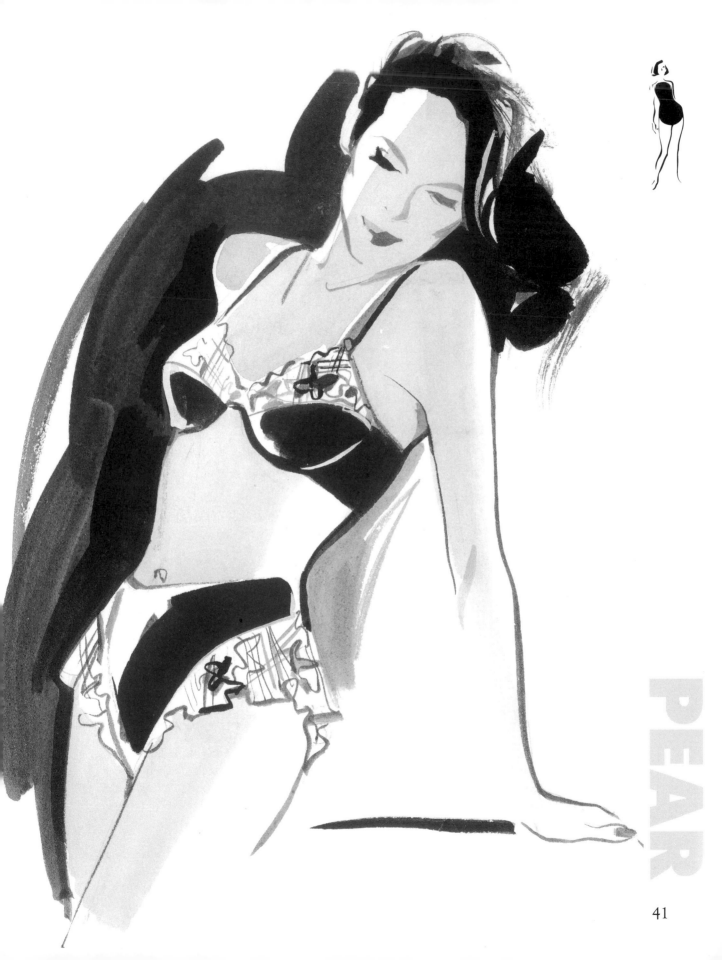

PEAR

41

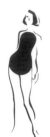

WEEK THREE
Your diet

This week can be a danger week. I found with my volunteer dieters that this was when they could lose heart. Weight loss, having been really good in the first two weeks, now tends to slow down. Boredom or resentment at not being able to indulge in your favourite high calorie foods may ambush all your good efforts so far.

If you are beginning to feel really miserable without some favourite but calorie-rich food, like salami, chocolate, or a piece of rich cake, then reward yourself—just once—with a small portion of what you crave. But make sure you really do savour and enjoy it. Don't feel guilty. Look on it as a treat, not the beginning of your total breakdown, and get on with the diet as strictly as before.

An occasional treat, say once a week, will do this body type absolutely no harm. (With my Rectangle body type, on the other hand, once I start eating, the brakes are off and I can't stop, so treats for my shape have to be strictly non-calorific.) However, from talking to clients and from the evidence of my questionnaire, I have found that chocolate cravings can be a real problem for some people, especially pre-menstrually. If you're in the stage of miserable craving, I think it is better to find a sensible way of dealing with this and I suggest that you try a low-calorie chocolate drink (most of the leading brands are making one) as a safe substitute rather than demolish a box of chocolates. This drink tastes chocolatey, gives you a feeling of fullness and comfort and gets rid of that awful sense of deprivation. But don't become addicted to this instead!

DAY FIFTEEN

Breakfast
One piece of fruit, cup of tea or coffee, skimmed milk from daily allowance.

Lunch
150 g (5 oz) cottage cheese with one chopped-up apple and orange, piece of wholemeal bread, cup of tea.

Supper
175 g (6 oz) white fish, grilled or steamed, green salad (as much as you like), low-cal dressing (either commercial brand or home-made (see recipe, page 72), 150 g (5oz) low-fat fruit yogurt.

DAY SIXTEEN

Breakfast
Same as above.

Lunch
Two hard-boiled eggs chopped into large mixed salad (from permitted vegetables), low-cal dressing (see recipe, page 72), cup of tea.

Supper
Vegetable casserole (see recipe, page 73), wholemeal bread or roll, two-fruit salad and 15 ml (1 tbsp) low-fat natural yogurt.

DAY SEVENTEEN

Breakfast
Same as above.

Lunch
Baked potato with low-cal coleslaw or homemade with creamy low-cal dressing (see recipe, page 72), 150 g (5 oz) pot of low-fat fruit yogurt, cup of tea.

Supper
100 g (4 oz) fresh or tinned salmon, steamed vegetables (from permitted vegetables), fresh fruit salad (from permitted fruit).

DAY EIGHTEEN

Breakfast
Same as above.

Lunch
150 g (5 oz) cottage cheese, green salad with olives, radishes and spring onions, low-cal dressing (see recipe, page 72), apple, cup of tea.

Supper
Spaghetti with broccoli (see recipe, page 74), baked pepper salad (see recipe, page 77), slice of wholemeal bread, banana split (1 tbsp iced vanilla yogurt instead of ice cream).

PEAR

Your exercise programme

Add this floor exercise to the three you're already doing.

Stomach clincher

1 Sit on the floor, legs wide apart and arms straight out at your sides at shoulder level.
2 Slowly bend forward and twist to the right, trying to touch your right knee with your forehead. Don't worry if you can't do this at the first attempt—as you become more supple you will get closer and closer. At the same time, slowly slide your left hand down your right leg, reaching as far towards (or beyond) your foot as you can. Stretch your right arm out behind you.
3 Return slowly to the starting position and repeat, taking your forehead to touch your left leg.
REPEAT WHOLE EXERCISE FIVE TIMES.

EXERCISE REPETITIONS: WEEK THREE	
Whole Leg Toner	3
Hip and Thigh Toner	3
Stomach and Waist Trimmer	4
Stomach Clincher	5

DAY NINETEEN
Breakfast
Same as above.
Lunch
Pitta bread spread with 50g (2 oz) hummus, sliced tomatoes, lettuce; 150g (5 oz) low-fat natural yogurt with one piece of fruit chopped in, cup of tea.
Supper
Quarter chicken roasted, steamed or grilled, big salad or selection of vegetables from permitted list, baked apple with 1 tsp honey and 1 tbsp frozen yogurt.

DAY TWENTY
Breakfast
Same as above.
Lunch
150 g (5 oz) low-fat natural yogurt, two pieces fruit chopped in, sprinkling of sunflower seeds (optional).
Supper
Salade Niçoise (see recipe, page 76), wholemeal bread, glass unsweetened fruit juice.

DAY TWENTY-ONE
Breakfast
Same as above
Lunch
Baked potato, creamy low-cal dressing (see recipe, page 72), baked pepper and anchovy (see recipe, page 77), one piece of fruit, cup of tea.
Supper
150 g (5 oz) white fish baked, steamed or grilled, two tomatoes and one medium onion, sliced onto lettuce, low-cal dressing (see recipe, page 72), small bunch of grapes.

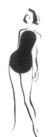

WEEK FOUR
Positive action: start at the top

JUST AS clothes with curves suit a Pear-type woman best, so do soft, wavy and not too short hairstyles. But do treat yourself to a good cut with a hair stylist who will take into consideration the weight and wave of your own hair and the shape of your face.

If you want to change the colour of your hair, bear in mind that its natural tone is the one which suits your skin and eye colour best. Unless you are aiming for a dramatic look (dark-haired Madonna was never meant to be a blonde), keep within your natural colour range. Dramatic colour changes can look sensational when you're young (and can afford an expensive professional style—and its maintenance), but they are hardening and ageing to older skins.

Professionally done high- and low-lights can be the most flattering way of adding zing to your hair without clashing with the rest of your colouring. But it can be expensive. I always say that if you had to choose, a good cut is the priority. Your own hair colour, glossy and healthy on this diet, will then look as exciting as can be.

PEAR

44

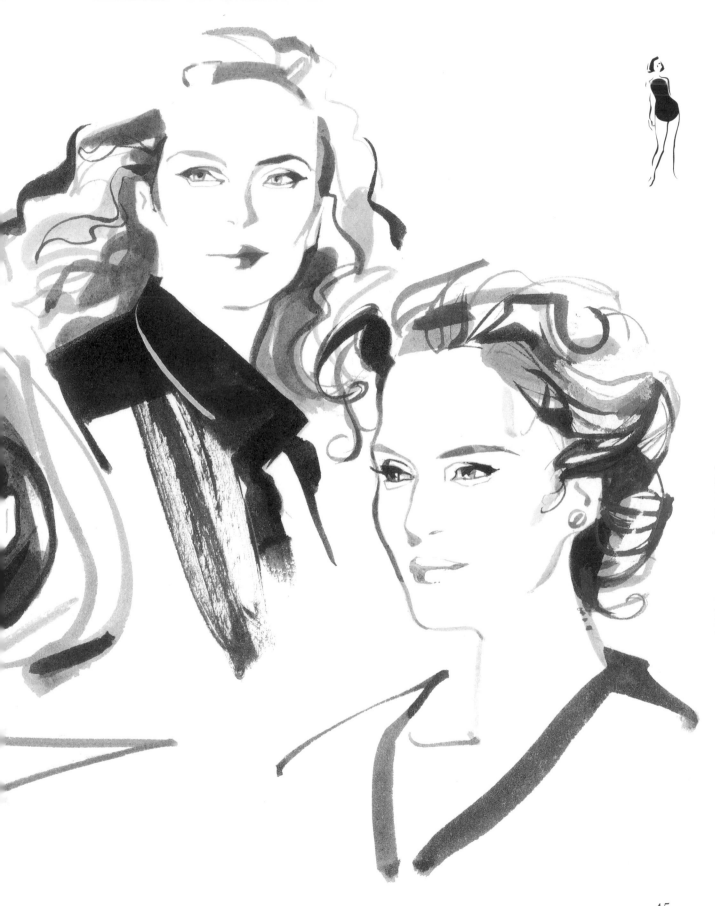

45

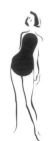

WEEK FOUR
Your diet

You are over the danger period of that third week. Although you may be disappointed that the scales do not register quite as much loss as you hoped I'm sure that by now you are feeling so much better—both slimmer and fitter—that you are quite happy to enter your fourth week. If Week Three had marked a plateau in your weight loss, then by the end of this fourth week I am pretty certain you will find you have lost *more* than you hoped.

DAY TWENTY-TWO
Breakfast
One piece of fruit, cup of tea or coffee, skimmed milk from your daily allowance.
Lunch
Two-egg omelette with mixed herbs, green beans and carrots, or any two vegetables from the permitted list, 150 g (5 oz) low-fat fruit yogurt, cup of tea.
Supper
100 g (4 oz) peeled prawns, large mixed salad, creamy low-cal dressing (see recipe, page 72), wholemeal bread, two-fruit salad, 1 tbsp frozen yogurt.

DAY TWENTY-THREE
Breakfast
Same as above.

'I feel much better altogether. I'm not eating anything unnecessary. I feel much more like making love to my husband now and feel much less of a lump.'

JB

Lunch
100 g (4 oz) cottage cheese with apple and orange chopped in, wholemeal bread, cup of tea.
Supper
Ratatouille (see recipe, page 74), 50 g (2 oz) brown rice, green salad, low-cal dressing (see recipe, page 72), piece of fruit

DAY TWENTY-FOUR
Breakfast
Same as above.
Lunch
Baked potato, 1 tbsp hummus, mixed salad, low-cal dressing (see recipe, page 72), 150 g (5 oz) low-fat fruit yogurt, cup of tea.
Supper
175 g (6 oz) chicken breast, rubbed with 1 tsp olive oil and herbs, grilled, selection of vegetables from permitted list, baked apple with 1 tsp honey and 1 tbsp low-fat natural yogurt

DAY TWENTY-FIVE
Breakfast
Same as above.
Lunch
300 ml (½ pt) any non-creamy packet soup, or homemade vegetable soup (see recipe, page 75), one piece wholemeal bread/toast, banana, cup of tea.
Supper
Mushroom and pepper risotto (see recipe, page 78), small green salad, low-cal dressing (see recipe, page 72), two-fruit salad.

DAY TWENTY-SIX
Breakfast
Same as above.
Lunch
100 g (4 oz) cottage cheese, baked pepper salad (see recipe, page 77), one piece of fruit, cup of tea.
Supper
Seafood pasta (see recipe, page 74), green salad, low-cal dressing (see recipe, page 72), one piece of fruit.

PEAR

Celebration treat:
buy something RED

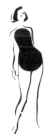

You've got there. Four weeks of a new way of eating and an exercise programme both of which are tailor-made for your body type and I hope you are really feeling more energetic, more attractive, more *you*. To celebrate, I would like to suggest that you go and buy yourself something red. It can be anything from a red scarf or handkerchief to red earrings, a jersey or—if you're feeling really triumphant—a red dress.

But remember, there are many shades of red. There are blue reds and orange reds; clear bright reds or muted, blended reds; light or deep reds. Before buying yourself your red treat, hold it under your chin to check that it is a flattering red for *you*. The right red will give you a healthy glow, and your skin, hair and eyes will look more vibrant. The wrong red will make you look pale and washed out. Any blemishes and dark shadows on your face are emphasized by the wrong colours.

Red is a marvellous colour. It lifts the spirits. It makes a definite statement; not 'poor little over-weight mousy me, please let me pass by, unseen in the crowd', but rather, 'I AM FULL OF LIFE! I AM CONFIDENT, I AM HAPPY, LOOK AT ME!'

DAY TWENTY-SEVEN

Breakfast
Same as above.
Lunch
Tabbouleh (see recipe, page 77) in wholemeal pitta bread, cup of tea.
Supper
150 g (5 oz) smoked haddock, steamed or poached in skimmed milk and water, two or more vegetables from permitted list, one piece of fruit cut up into 150 g (5 oz) low-fat natural yogurt.

DAY TWENTY-EIGHT

Breakfast
Same as above.
Lunch
Three fruits from permitted list made into fruit salad with 100g (4 oz) low-fat natural yogurt, cup of tea.
Supper
Quarter of chicken, grilled or dry roasted, large mixed salad, low-cal dressing (see recipe, page 72), wholemeal roll, one piece of fruit.

Your exercise programme

You can now increase the repetitions of your floor exercises as shown in the box below. I hope that by now you have also established a routine of walking, yoga, cycling, or exercise class or video at least twice a week and are really seeing the benefits of toned-up muscles, extra weight loss and improved circulation and spirits. You should be able to work out a pattern of exercise which will be easy and pleasurable to follow in the long term. Here's to a fitter, happier you!

EXERCISE REPETITIONS: WEEK FOUR	
Whole Leg Toner	4
Hip and Thigh Toner	4
Stomach and Waist Trimmer	5
Stomach Clincher	7

PEAR

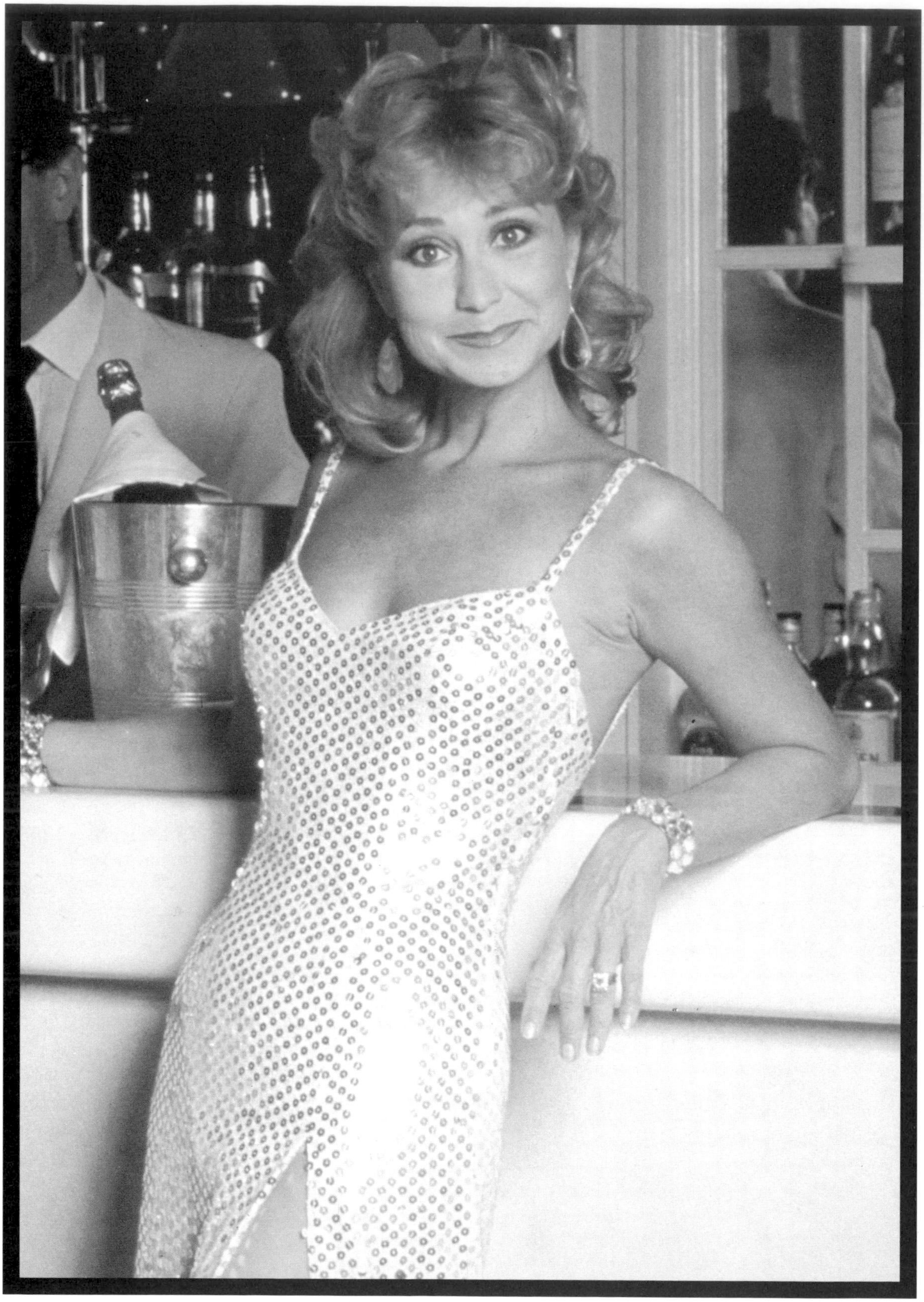

HOURGLASS TYPE
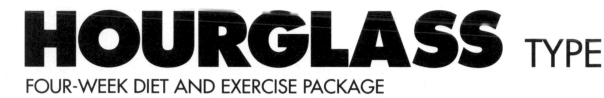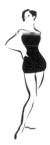

FOUR-WEEK DIET AND EXERCISE PACKAGE

THIS IS a four-week package of diet menus and exercise programme tailor-made for your body type and metabolism. A team of volunteer dieters tested this diet and exercise programme for six weeks, some for three months and more. Their experiences and comments went into improving it for you. With each week, my volunteer dieters and I found it was very encouraging to have a treat, or 'positive action', to lift our spirits and keep us going into next week. As you read through the package you will see what I mean.

Individual characteristics

The Hourglass type has a volatile energy level which can be sabotaged by bad eating habits (this type is particularly prone to snacking) and too much caffeine/alcohol. All this can result in swings of energy, often leaving her feeling exhausted and heading for the sofa.

The Hourglass-type's diet and exercise regime should introduce regularity and moderation into her life and so meals are equally balanced, three times a day. Nibbling and snacking are discouraged, and regular but not too strenuous exercise is suggested. This is a physically balanced type of body with a natural grace and poise and so exercises which strengthen the body and enhance suppleness and grace are particularly suitable, eg. yoga, Callanetics, tennis, brisk walking and swimming.

The Hourglass type will lose weight best and feel most happy and energetic (and therefore more likely to stick to the regime), if she eats a moderate amount of low-fat protein, such as chicken, fish and cottage cheese, and plenty of fruit and raw or lightly-cooked vegetables.

Felicity Kendal is a classic Hourglass. Her whole look is curvy, rather than angular. She has a balanced body; shoulders and hips of equal width and she has a pronounced waist. Her tummy is flattish and her hips and thighs curvy rather than straight. The dress, with its scoop neckline, suits her. Although the bodice seaming is rather too straight for her body line, the fabric is fluid and clingy and so follows her shape. Her hair style too is suitably soft and wavy. She is a woman who knows how to dress and make the most of herself.

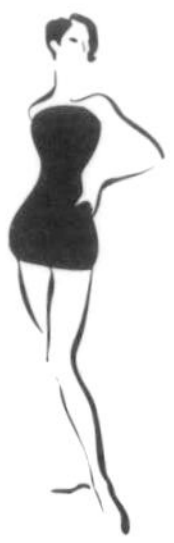

HOURGLASS-TYPE WEIGHT AND MEASUREMENTS BEFORE DIETING, AND SIX WEEKS LATER

	WEIGHT (kg/st & lbs)		MEASUREMENTS (cms/ins)					
				BEFORE			AFTER	
NAME	BEFORE	AFTER	BUST	WAIST	HIPS	BUST	WAIST	HIPS
Alix	72.5/11 7	68.5/10 12	94/37¾	75/30	102.5/41	92.5/37	74/29½	92.5/37
Lindsay	74/11 10	66/10 6	97.5/39	81/32½	109/43½	92.5/37	76/30½	104/40½
Margaret	101/16 1	93.5/14 12	111/44½	104/40½	124/49½	109/43½	91/36½	115/46
Nicky	153.5/24 5	146/23 2	160/64	145/58	165/66	145/58	141/56½	162.5/65
Denise	73/11 9	67/10 9	104/41½	82.5/33	107.5/43	96/38½	79/31½	104/40½
Anne	85.5/13 8	80.5/12 11	102/40¾	87.5/35	116/46½	95.5/38¼	84/33½	109/43½
Caroline	62/9 12	57/9 0	87.5/35	72.5/29	97.5/39	82/32¾	69/27½	94/37½
Clare	81/12 12	78/12 6	101/40½	82.5/33	115/46	94.5/37¾	80/32	109/43½
Andrea	57.5/9 2	54/8 8	85.5/34¼	67.5/27	91/36½	85/34	64/25½	86/34½
Sonia	67/10 9	63/10 0	100/40	70/28	100/40	95/38	67.5/27	95/38

The Hourglass-type is a balanced body type who puts on weight equally on top and bottom. As was expected, our volunteer dieters in this group lost their weight in equal proportion.

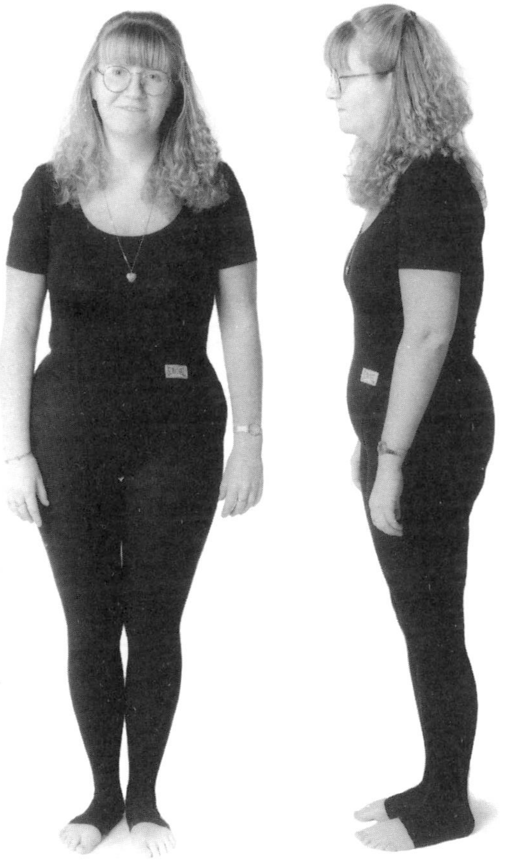

BEFORE

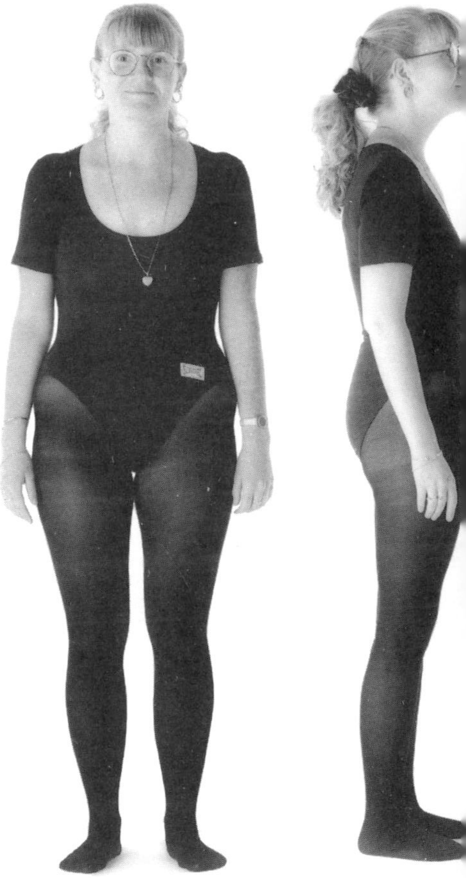

AFTER

Our volunteer above lost a tremendous 8 kg (18 lbs) in six weeks, with 5 cms (2 ins) off her bust, 5 cms (2 ins) from her waist and 7.5 cms (3 ins) from her hips.

She has lost weight all over—her face, upper chest, back, arms and legs are also noticeable thinner, giving a total refinement of shape.

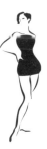

HOURGLASS-TYPE DIETERS WEIGHT LOSS OVER SIX WEEKS (kgs/lbs)

NAME	WEEK:	1	2	3	4	5	6	TOTAL WEIGHT LOSS
Alix		3.1/7	0/0	0.5/1	1.4/3	+0.5/1	+0.5/1	− 4/9
Lindsay		2.2/5	0.9/2	0.5/1	1.8/4	0/0	2.7/6	− 8/18
Margaret		3.5/8	0.9/2	1.8/4	0.9/2	0.5/1	0/0	−7.5/17
Nicky		2/4½	0.9/2	2/4½	0.9/2	0.5/1	1.4/3	−7.5/17
Denise		0.9/2	0.5/1	1.4/3	1.4/3	1.4/3	0.9/2	−6.3/14
Anne		0.9/2	0.9/2	+1.8/4	1.4/3	2.2/5	1.4/3	− 5/11
Caroline		2/4½	0.9/2	0.5/1	0.5/1	0.7/1½	0.9/2	−5.5/12
Clare		0.9/2	0.5/1	0/0	0.5/1	0.5/1	0.5/1	−2.7/6
Andrea		1.4/3	+0.5/1	0.9/2	1.4/3	0.9/2	+0.5/1	−3.6/8
Sonia		0.9/2	1.8/4	0.5/1	0.5/1	0.5/1	0/0	− 4/9

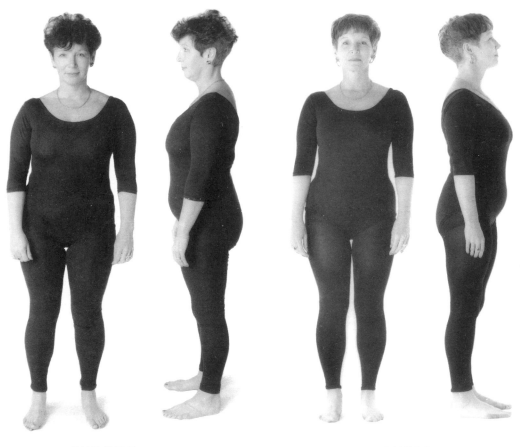

BEFORE　　　　　　　　　　**AFTER**

Our volunteer, above, who lost a total of 6.3 kg (14 lbs) in the six weeks, lost 7.5 cms (3 ins) from her bust, 3.75 cms (1½ ins) from her waist and 6 cms (2½ ins) from her hips. Before she began, she was concerned that her face would become gaunt as on previous diets. She was delighted that although she lost so much weight, her face did not get thin and drawn.

It is interesting how this weight loss has made this volunteer more of an Hourglass by refining the whole central area of her torso.

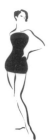

WEEK ONE
Positive action: enhance your style

AS YOU'VE already seen, we don't all share the same body shape and a particular style of clothing that looks fantastic on one woman can look dreadful on somebody else. And this is not just a matter of slenderness. Wearing clothes which suit your body shape, drawing attention to your good points and hiding your not so good, can give you the appearance of having *lost 3 kg (7 lbs)* before you even begin your diet.

The basic principle of style is that you wear clothes which have the same or similar line to your body line. The Hourglass is the classic female shape; Brigitte Bardot, Marilyn Monroe, Naomi Campbell and Julia Roberts are obvious Hourglasses; Dame Judi Dench, Dawn French and Oprah Winfrey more curvy versions. As an Hourglass, when you are slim you have the widest range of styles to choose from. Put a slim Hourglass in a straight skirt, better suited to the Rectangle or Triangle types, and she looks sexy, sexier than the two angular types because the skirt emphasizes her curves.

Put a slim Hourglass in a pair of masculine-style jeans and she doesn't look workmanlike, as if these straight trousers were made for her, as a slim Rectangle would, but her curvy hips and pronounced waist make her look like a woman emphasizing her *difference* from the cowboys for whom such clothes were originally made.

For the most flattering dressing, and credibility in business, however, the Hourglass looks best in clothes which follow her body line rather than over-emphasizing her curves. Jackets and tops should be slightly waisted and curve gently over her hips. Belts look good on this shape. Keep all fabrics light and soft, wool crêpes, linen, silk, suede—nothing too crisp and uniform-like.

Skirts, trousers and shorts are all more flattering to this shape if they have a few soft pleats easing from the waistband over the hips. The tulip-shape skirt with a short curvy jacket is an excellent smart profile for the Hourglass body type.

Like the Pear, however, the greater domination of female hormones in this type means this is a shape which can quite easily put on weight. But unlike the Pear, this type puts weight on pretty much equally on the hips and bust. Although when slim this is the easiest shape to dress, when the Hourglass is substantially overweight she can have a lot of problems choosing what style of clothes to wear. Carrying a few stones extra (think of Liz Taylor at her curviest), the Hourglass can feel she's more like a Cottage Loaf.

I always tell my Hourglass clients that if I (a Rectangle) ever had another life I'd ask to come back as an Hourglass, but a slim one.

Generally speaking then, all detail on clothes or accessories should be curved rather than angular, soft, rounded shoulder pads, rounded lapels, oval belt buckles and not too boxy handbags.

If you're young, or young-at-heart, and don't have to dress for business then you may like to try what the actress and comedienne Dawn French looks so good in, a large oversize jumper in a good colour and bold pattern over black leggings or tapered trousers.

The Hourglass will often have narrow ankles and pretty feet and it is a good idea to draw attention to them with good shoes and ankle boots.

If you are very overweight

If this is the case these general style pointers need a bit of modification. There is a tendency for overweight women to try to camouflage everything and some end up wearing a tent in despair. But all shapes, even carrying a lot of extra weight, still have their distinctive good points and clothes should show these to advantage.

The Hourglass is a balanced body type and this means that when she puts on a lot of weight she is heavier all over, but most noticeably in the bust and hips. She will still keep her waist but may feel uncomfortable in waisted, fitted clothes because they emphasize her curves too much. She may, therefore, feel happier in softly draped, longer jackets which have straighter lines, over fluid, gathered or pleated skirts.

I would suggest that you still emphasize your

HOURGLASS

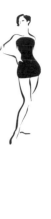

waist a little under your jacket, with a belt perhaps. But although your jackets might be straighter make sure they are in a soft fabric, like a washed silk, so that they neither look like a uniform nor are shapeless on you. Keep your shoulder pads rounded rather than straight, they help balance the hippiness of your shape when you put on a lot of extra pounds.

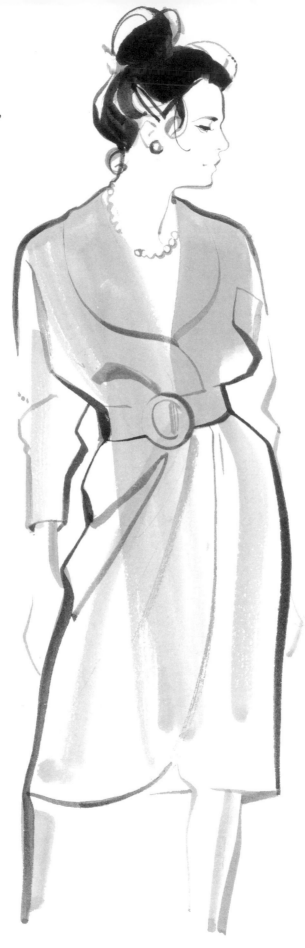

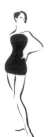

WEEK ONE

Jewellery

Jewellery for the Hourglass follows the same line as her body and her clothes. Keep detail predominantly curvy with a little geometrical shape for a change. Necklaces are prettier on you if they are beads or the rounder-linked chains rather than those more severe metal collars or torques which are fashionable. Pearls really look fantastic on the Hourglass and the Pear.

With brooches, again you should keep to a largely swept, curved line, with a few straight lines for contrast. But remember, *scale* is as important in jewellery as it is in clothes. It has to be the right size for you. If you are large boned (as a rough guide, if your wrist measures 16.5cms [6½ins] or more) then

your jewellery pieces ought to be large and important. If you are medium (14–16.5cms [5½–6½ins]) to small boned (less than 14cms [5½ins]) then make sure your jewellery is not too heavy and of smaller scale so that it doesn't overwhelm you.

Watches should have round or oval faces and unless you are large boned be careful that they are not too big and their straps not too heavy.

So, as your first positive action, make yourself look slimmer and boost your morale by wearing the right clothes and accessories for your shape. Then start on Week One of your tailor-made diet and exercise plan and begin to lose pounds of real weight. Begin today to realize the true potential of your shape.

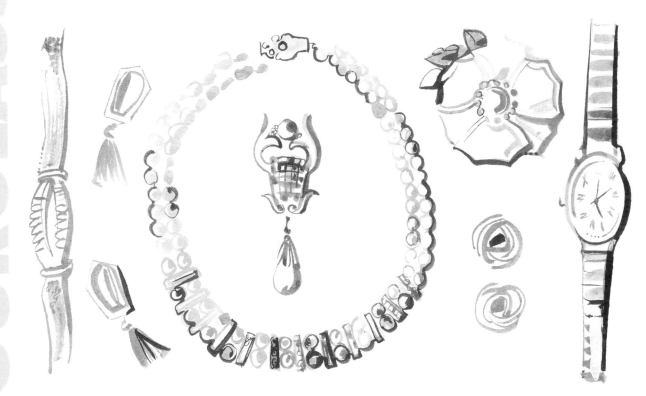

HOURGLASS

Starting your diet

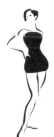

This is a low-fat diet. With a reduced fat, reduced sugar and increased fibre intake, this diet takes into account the latest findings on healthy nutrition. There is a good deal of evidence that the Hourglass type particularly thrives on a diet high in raw fruit and vegetables with protein and carbohydrate from unrefined sources in equal balance.

The menus which follow are for those of you who like a structured diet. For the rest, they are suggestions for meals based on the basic principles of your body-type diet of low-fat protein (like cottage cheese or white fish), unrefined carbohydrates (like baked potato, wholemeal bread, brown rice), with almost limitless salad and vegetables, and generous amounts of fruit. The Hourglass type's metabolism responds best to three balanced meals a day, definitely including a breakfast. She should resist nibbling in between meals, although she is allowed permitted vegetables or one piece of fruit as emergency gap fillers during the day.

You can switch meals around from day to day or repeat easy or favourite ones—as long as you have one breakfast, one lunch meal and one supper meal every day. And *no snacking*. Useful, though not ideal, if you are too busy, or disinclined to cook, are the ready-made, low-calorie frozen meals. You may substitute these for your main meal but add a salad or some slightly cooked vegetables. This diet should not only help you to lose weight but to be healthier, look better and feel great.

This diet does not allow for alcohol. There are two main reasons for this: alcohol represents empty calories and I would rather you got food value for your extra calories in the shape of an extra piece of fruit, or another helping of salad or vegetables or even a slightly larger helping of protein: fish or eggs or chicken. But most importantly, alcohol undermines our self-control—and can be addictive. Once we've had one drink it's much easier to have another, and then our resolve goes and we're eating anything that comes our way.

It's much easier and generally more efficient if you can cut out alcohol for the duration of your diet. Many women find that they can lose weight just by doing this, so unaware were they of how many extra calories they were consuming every day in liquid form.

However, I am aware that for some women this is an impossibility and if it is the difference between going on the diet or not, obviously I would rather

---

DAILY ALLOWANCE

300ml (½ pt) skimmed milk
15 g (½ oz) low-fat spread

Beverages: try to keep your intake of tea/coffee to two cups a day, but drink plenty of water and have as many cups of herb tea as you like

Unlimited vegetables (preferably raw, otherwise boiled/steamed):

asparagus	aubergine	bean sprouts	beetroot
broccoli	brussel sprouts	cabbage	carrots
cauliflower	celery	chard	chicory
courgettes	cucumbers	French beans	endive
escarole	green/red pepper	kale	lettuce
mange-tout peas	mushrooms	okra	onions
parsley	radishes	runner beans	spinach
spring greens	tomatoes	turnips	watercress

One piece of fruit extra to meal allowances:

apple	apricot	handful blackberries	grapefruit
kiwi	nectarine	orange	peach
pear	plum	tangerine	watermelon, 1 slice

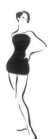

WEEK ONE

you follow the dieting guidelines and limit your alcohol to one drink a day, preferably with your meal.

For vegetarians there are recipes for main meal substitutions in the recipe supplement on pages 72–9.

DAY ONE

Breakfast
Half grapefruit (or other fruit from permitted list), 25 g (1 oz) museli, bran flakes, puffed wheat or any other unsweetened cereal (with skimmed milk from daily allowance), cup of tea or coffee.

Lunch
150 g (5 oz) cottage cheese with one chopped-up apple and orange, piece of wholemeal bread or toast (with low-fat spread from daily allowance), cup of tea. (Many Hourglass-type dieters find this the perfect lunch for them. You may choose to have it most days instead of the other suggestions.)

Supper
Quarter chicken roasted, steamed or grilled, big salad, low-cal dressing (see recipe, page 72) or selection of vegetables from permitted list, baked apple with 1 tsp honey and 1 tbsp frozen yogurt.

DAY TWO

Breakfast
1 egg, poached, boiled or scrambled, one piece of toast (with low-fat spread from daily allowance), cup of tea or coffee.

Lunch
300 ml (½ pt) any non-creamy packet soup, or homemade vegetable soup (see recipe, page 75), wholemeal roll, 150 g (5 oz) low-fat natural yogurt with one piece of fruit chopped in, cup of tea.

Supper
100 g (4 oz) fresh or tinned salmon, steamed vegetables (from permitted vegetables), fresh fruit salad (from permitted fruit).

DAY THREE

Breakfast
Either as Day 1 or Day 2.

Lunch
Pitta bread spread with 50 g (2 oz) hummus, sliced tomatoes, lettuce; 150 g (5 oz) low-fat natural yogurt with one piece of fruit, cup of tea.

Supper
Salade Niçoise (see recipe, page 76), wholemeal bread, two-fruit salad, 1 tbsp low-fat natural yogurt.

DAY FOUR

Breakfast
Either as Day 1 or Day 2.

Lunch
150 g (5 oz) cottage cheese mixed with chopped olives, radishes, spring onions, green salad, one piece wholemeal bread (with low-fat spread from daily allowance), apple, cup of tea.

Supper
Spaghetti with broccoli (see recipe, page 74), baked pepper salad (see recipe, page 77), banana split (1 tbsp iced yogurt instead of ice cream).

DAY FIVE

Breakfast
As Day 1.

Lunch
1 hard-boiled egg, 25 g (1 oz) feta cheese chopped into large mixed salad (from permitted vegetables), creamy low-cal dressing (see recipe, page 72), one piece of wholemeal bread toasted (with low-fat spread from daily allowance) as croutons, cup of tea.

Supper
Vegetable casserole (see recipe, page 73), 50 g (2 oz) rice (dried weight, preferably brown) boiled, salad of green pepper and onion chopped in rings, low-cal dressing (see recipe, page 72), one piece of fruit.

DAY SIX

Breakfast
Either as Day 1 or Day 2.

Lunch
150 g (5 oz) low-fat natural yogurt or 100 g

HOURGLASS

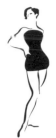

(4 oz) fromage frais (8% fat), two pieces of fruit chopped in, sprinkling of sunflower seeds (optional).

Supper
100 g (4 oz) peeled prawns, large mixed salad, creamy low-cal dressing (see recipe, page 72), one slice of wholemeal bread, two-fruit salad, 1 tbsp frozen yogurt.

DAY SEVEN

Breakfast
Either as Day 1 or Day 2.

Lunch
Baked potato, 110g (4 oz) baked beans, large green salad, low-cal dressing (see recipe, page 72), one piece of fruit, cup of tea.

Supper
150 g (5 oz) white fish baked, steamed or grilled, two tomatoes and one medium onion, sliced onto lettuce, low-cal dressing (see recipe, page 72), small bunch of grapes.

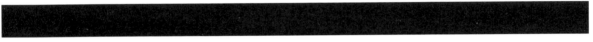

❛I've always been quite good at losing weight but as I got older (I'm now 56) it got harder and harder and I found myself just putting weight on. I thought I would have to resign myself to being a pudding for the rest of my life. And then my daughter Lindsay [one of the volunteers] gave me your diet and everything you said about the Hourglass type was so true of me I thought this might be a diet that would really work for me.

I didn't lose any weight for the first fortnight, although I felt much better and *slimmer*, but I persevered because the food suited me so well and was healthier than what I had been eating. Then I lost 2.7 kg (6 lbs) and I have found that I tend to follow this fortnightly pattern. Now I know about it I don't worry. I've lost over 12.5 kg (2 stone) and want to carry on for another 6.3 kg (1 stone). I am so delighted with it all.

The cottage cheese lunch is marvellous. As I work I just take it to work with me and I even have it at weekends sometimes, I like it so much.

Thank you so much for a lovely diet. I've got back the figure I thought I'd lost for ever!❜

Coral

HOURGLASS

57

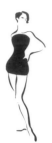

WEEK ONE
Your exercise programme

The Hourglass type is attracted to exercise that is not too energetic; road running and squash are seldom their first choice in an attempt to get fit. But tennis, swimming, walking and dancing are all more suited to their physical body type and temperament and I hope that you will be able to organize yourself into exercising two or three times a week; swimming for half an hour at a time, or walking briskly to work, or on a long country hike at the weekend, or spending an evening dancing.

Although the Hourglass type does not need to work out hard in order to feel fit and happy, any exercise helps a dieter lose weight by using up extra calories (a relatively energetic half-hour of tennis burns 210 calories), and by increasing the basic metabolic rate for a few hours after the exercise has ceased.

There is also a 'feel good' factor to exercising which cannot be over-emphasized. If you're doing the exercise that suits your body type and disposition it undoubtedly lifts the spirits, makes you generally more positive about yourself, and more in tune with your body. You will become increasingly less likely to neglect and abuse it.

A medium- to low-impact aerobics class or yoga, or both, will really improve your body tone and rate of weight loss. So if you can increase your weekly exercise quota to at least two half-hour episodes I know you will improve the efficiency of the diet and your feeling of well-being. I also include three floor exercises to be done every day to strengthen and tone the stomach, thighs and hips. Good Luck.

Waist twister

This floor exercise tones up the waist, tummy and sides of your torso without putting any strain on your back.

1 Lie flat on the floor, with the small of your back pressed into the floor. Stretch arms above head and point toes, making yourself as tall as possible.
2 Clasp your hands behind your head. Lift your head and arms, keeping your elbows as open as possible, and look at your toes which should now be pulled towards you. Make your tummy muscles hold you in this position. *Do not pull on your neck. Hold position while you count to ten.*
3 Slowly relax your position until you are lying flat again with hands still behind your head.
4 Bend your right leg and lift your knee to your body. Lift head and arms and twist your torso so that the left elbow comes as close as possible to touching the right knee.
5 Relax and lie flat and then repeat Step 4 again, four more times.
6 Relax and then repeat the whole exercise with the opposite leg and elbow.

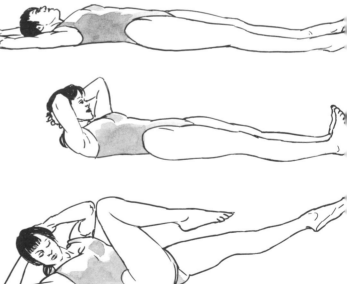

HOURGLASS

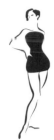

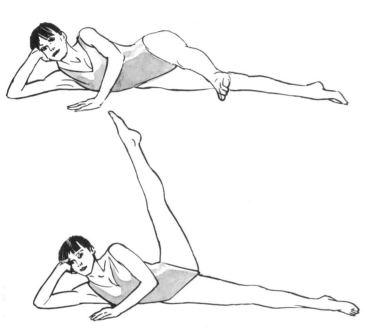

Hip and thigh toner

This will involve the muscles which run from your hips and down the outside edge of your thighs. Again keep your body in a straight line during the whole exercise.

1 Lie on your right side, supporting your head with your right arm, both legs straight.

2 Slowly raise both legs a few inches off the floor, keeping them as straight as possible. *Hold the position while you count to five.* Then lower.

3 Keeping your body in a straight line raise your left leg into the air until it is at a right angle to your hip.

4 Slowly lower it across your body, keeping your leg straight, and with your foot as close to shoulder level as possible. *Hold your extended foot just above ground level and count to five.*

5 Raise your leg again into the air and return it to the starting position.

6 Raise both legs off floor. *Hold the position while you count to 30.* Lower legs to floor.

7 Turn over and repeat the whole exercise with your other leg.

REPEAT EXERCISE TWO TIMES.

Thigh shaper

This will make your thighs ache, particularly the under-used muscles that run along the top side, but just think how they will be improving in tone, strength and shape every time you do it.

1 Stand sideways to a chair or table, feet a hip-width apart, and rest your hand on it to balance yourself (no desperate gripping to save your thigh muscles having to work).

2 Raise yourself up on tip-toe and then slowly squat as low as possible. Do not, however, allow your hips to be nearer the ground than your knees and keep your back ram-rod straight.

3 Raise yourself about 15cms (6ins) and hold while you count to three and then slowly return to your base position.

REPEAT EXERCISE TEN TIMES.

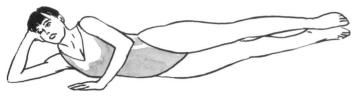

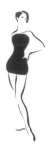

WEEK TWO
Positive action: instant healthy glow

GO AND buy yourself a blusher. Nothing lifts the contours of the face and the colour of a complexion more immediately and naturally than blusher. Buy a powder in a neutral rosy tone and apply it as shown in the illustration below.

1 Brush blush along the cheekbone, starting on a level with the outer edge of your iris and feathering it upwards and outwards as far as the hairline at the top of your ear.

2 You might like also to add the slightest touch of colour to your temples and chin.

3 Blend the edges with a soft powder brush. Never have definite lines in any make-up you apply.

Many women say to me they don't use make-up which usually means they are not confident about using it and don't like a made-up look. My answer is that from our mid-twenties onwards our colouring begins to fade and the definition of our features softens with age. I never advocate a stagey effect, but do point out that if you are in business well-applied make-up gives your features greater definition and adds more authority to your whole image.

If you still feel reluctant or lacking in competence, try using just your new blusher and a soft neutral lipstick and see if you like the effect. This should make your complexion brighter, your eyes more intense in colour and your face more contoured.

HOURGLASS

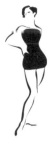

Subtly applied eye make-up needs a bit more technique and practice. But it is eye make-up which most fair-skinned, light-eyelashed women particularly feel they need most. In my classes, even the most tentative women manage a professional job after experimenting for half an hour. Without being able to advise you personally, taking into account your individual colouring and shape of eye, I can only give the following steps as a general pointer.

By now you may well be noticing that your first week's dieting has begun to reveal more marked cheekbones and a cleaner jawline. There is nothing nicer than seeing your neck grow longer and your face begin to emerge finer and younger-looking. Certainly, on this diet your skin will improve, although you may find that during the first week it's a bit spotty as you clear some of the toxins out of your system. By the end it will be finer textured and glowing.

1 Highlighter: using an eyeshadow sponge, apply a light, neutral colour on the whole area of your upper eye from eyelid to brow.

2 Lid: apply a light to medium colour just on the lid (a taupe or soft olive suit most people), blending with a small brush.

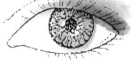

3 Orbital bone: apply a darker colour along the upper eye-socket crease, blending it onto the lid at the outer corner of the eye. Blend all the colours with a soft brush. The end result must look like a wash of colour over your lid, getting darker towards the socket and the outside edge. No stripes or hard edges please.

4 Mascara: finish the look off with a couple of coats of brown mascara on the upper lashes, and one coat on the lower.

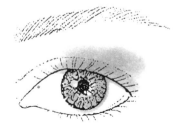

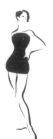

WEEK TWO
Your diet

HOURGLASS

DAY EIGHT
Breakfast
Half grapefruit (or other fruit from permitted list), 25 g (1 oz) muesli, bran flakes, puffed wheat, or other non-sweetened cereals (with skimmed milk from daily allowance), cup of tea or coffee.
Lunch
Tabbouleh (see recipe, page 77) in wholemeal pitta bread, grated carrot salad with orange juice as dressing, small bunch of grapes, cup of tea.
Supper
Mushroom omelette (see recipe, page 76), green beans and broccoli, or any two vegetables from permitted list, 150 g (5 oz) low-fat fruit yogurt.

DAY NINE
Breakfast
One egg, poached, boiled or scrambled, one piece of toast (with low-fat spread from daily allowance), cup of tea or coffee.
Lunch
100 g (4 oz) cottage cheese with apple and orange chopped in, one piece of wholemeal bread, cup of tea.
Supper
Ratatouille (see recipe, page 74) with 50 g (2 oz) rice (dried weight, preferably brown) boiled, one piece wholemeal bread, ginger bananas (see recipe, page 79).

DAY TEN
Breakfast
Either as Day 8 or Day 9.
Lunch
Baked potato with low-cal coleslaw or homemade with creamy low-cal dressing (see recipe, page 72), 150 g (5 oz) low-fat fruit yogurt, cup of tea.
Supper
175 g (6 oz) chicken breast, rubbed with 1 tsp olive oil and herbs, grilled, selection of vegetables from permitted list, baked apple with 1 tsp honey and 1 tbsp low-fat natural yogurt.

DAY ELEVEN
Breakfast
Either as Day 8 or Day 9.
Lunch
300 ml (½ pt) any non-creamy packet soup or homemade vegetable soup (see recipe, page75), one piece wholemeal bread/toast, banana, cup of tea.
Supper
175 g (6 oz) fresh (grilled) or tinned tuna (in brine not oil), large mixed salad, low-cal dressing (see recipe, page 72), fresh fruit salad (from permitted list), 1 tbsp low-fat natural yogurt.

DAY TWELVE
Breakfast
Either as Day 8 or Day 9.
Lunch
100 g (4 oz) cottage cheese, baked pepper salad (see recipe, page 77), one piece wholemeal bread or roll, one piece of fruit, cup of tea.
Supper
Seafood pasta (see recipe, page 74), green salad, low-cal dressing (see recipe, page 72), one piece of fruit.

'I have never before lost so much weight, and so quickly. I feel for the first time in my adult life that I can be a slim woman.'

Margaret

Your exercise programme

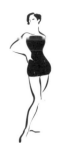

You should be beginning to feel lighter and fitter by now. I hope that you have managed to establish some sort of regular exercise programme, swimming or playing tennis at least twice a week, or going to an exercise class and increasing your activity level in your everyday life (walking to work, running up stairs, etc). Increase the repetitions of the floor exercises given you for the first week as outlined in the box below.

EXERCISE REPETITIONS: WEEK TWO	
Waist Twister	2
Hip and Thigh Toner	3
Thigh Shaper	15

DAY THIRTEEN

Breakfast
Either as Day 8 or Day 9.

Lunch
Baked pepper and anchovy (see recipe, page 77), one wholemeal pitta bread, 150 g (5 oz) low-fat fruit yogurt, cup of tea.

Supper
Quarter of chicken, grilled or dry roasted, broccoli, green beans (or other permitted vegetables) steamed or boiled, two-fruit salad with 1 tbsp low-fat yogurt (or frozen yogurt).

DAY FOURTEEN

Breakfast
Either as Day 8 or Day 9.

Lunch
Three fruits from permitted list made into fruit salad with 100g (4 oz) low-fat natural yogurt, 1 tbsp muesli stirred in, cup of tea.

Supper
Chick pea curry (see recipe, page 74), 25 g (1 oz) rice (dried weight, preferably brown) boiled, large green salad, low-cal dressing (see recipe, page 72), one piece of fruit.

'In a way, the diet's real success for me was the way it changed my attitude to exercise and made me much more aware of my shape rather than my weight. I have begun to exercise both more frequently and more energetically than before, and now swim and run two or three times a week, and also try and have a couple of sessions on exercise and toning tables.

I have noticed a real difference in my body shape, and feel much slimmer and fitter, though my overall weight loss was fairly low. I am also more careful than ever to wear clothes that emphasize my good points. Though I was disappointed only to lose 2.7 kg (6 lbs), I was delighted and surprised by my inch-loss. The principles of the diet encouraged me to rethink my eating and exercising habits.'

Clare

HOURGLASS

63

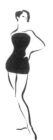

WEEK THREE
Positive action: good foundations

YOU ARE due for a reward for having got this far and lost those first pounds. Some of you may be as much as 3 kg (7 lbs) lighter by this point, others more like 1.8–2.3 kg (4–5 lbs). Whatever weight you have lost, you will notice a flattening of the bulges. Your waist will be more marked and your hips less fleshy. You may well feel like treating yourself to an indulgence that does not involve food. I suggest a glamorous piece of underwear as your treat which will make you feel pampered and proud of your curvy body.

Women with straight hips are more flattered by sporty underwear, but you—a woman with curvy hips and a waist—can get away with frilly, lacy underwear. A pretty underwired lace bra will make the most of your breasts and give you good support. Or if you're buying a pair of knickers, you can wear frilly French knickers or lace-trimmed bikinis. Or you may prefer to buy yourself a lace all-in-one. Make your choice and spoil yourself.

HOURGLASS

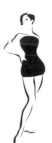

'This programme has made me really like my shape, I'm now proud to be curvy—instead of always wishing I had narrow hips. The style pointers have helped enormously (I've bought myself some good belts) and I don't feel I'm on a diet at all—except I keep on losing weight!'

Tricia

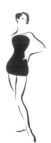

WEEK THREE
Your diet

This week can be a danger week. I found with my volunteer dieters that this could be the week when they lost heart. Weight loss may have been really good in the first two weeks but now it could slow down. You've been so good and you're fed up to think how much further you have to go. Boredom or resentment at not being able to indulge in your favourite high calorie foods may ambush all your good efforts so far.

If you are beginning to feel really miserable without some favourite but calorie-rich food, like salami, chocolate, or a piece of cake, then reward yourself just once—with a small portion of whatever you crave. But make sure you really savour and enjoy it. Don't feel guilty. Look on it as an earned treat, not the beginning of a total breakdown, and get on with the diet as strictly as before. An occasional treat, say once a week, will do absolutely no harm.

Remember though, it's not absolutely necessary to eat the thing you crave. I have an Hourglass friend who says that *sniffing* the chocolate or salami or whatever she craves and *imagining herself eating it* is satisfying enough. Lucky her! But then the Pear and the Hourglass shapes tend to be more disciplined about food than the Rectangle (me). Once I start to eat, unless I have a dietary curb, I will eat until there's nothing left whether it's a delicious casserole or a box of Belgian chocolates. So these sort of treats are not ideal for me.

From talking to clients and from the evidence of my questionnaire, I have found that chocolate cravings can be a real problem for some people, especially pre-menstrually. If you find yourself in the stage of miserable craving, I think it is better to find a sensible way of dealing with this and I suggest that you try a low-calorie chocolate drink (most of the leading brands are making one) as a safer substitute than demolishing a box of chocolates. This drink tastes chocolatey, gives you a feeling of fullness and comfort and gets rid of that awful sense of deprivation. But don't go getting addicted to this instead!

DAY FIFTEEN
Breakfast
Half grapefruit (or other fruit from permitted list), 25 g (1 oz) muesli, bran flakes, puffed wheat or any other unsweetened cereal (with skimmed milk from daily allowance), cup of tea or coffee.
Lunch
150 g (5 oz) cottage cheese with one chopped-up apple and orange, piece of wholemeal bread or toast (with low-fat spread from daily allowance), cup of tea.
Supper
Quarter chicken roasted, steamed or grilled, big salad, low-cal dressing (see recipe, page 72) or selection of vegetables from permitted list, baked apple with 1 tsp honey and 1 tbsp frozen yogurt.

DAY SIXTEEN
Breakfast
1 egg, poached, boiled or scrambled, one piece of toast (with low-fat spread from daily allowance), cup tea or coffee.
Lunch
300 ml (½ pt) any non-creamy packet soup, or homemade vegetable soup (see recipe, page 75), wholemeal roll, 150 g (5 oz) low-fat natural yogurt with one piece of fruit chopped in, cup of tea.
Supper
100 g (4 oz) fresh or tinned salmon, steamed vegetables (from permitted vegetables), fresh fruit salad (from permitted fruit).

'It doesn't feel like a diet. I feel I can go on eating like this for good. I enjoy being innovative and making up new soups and salads.'

Alix

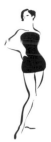

DAY SEVENTEEN

Breakfast
Either as Day 15 or Day 16.

Lunch
Pitta bread spread with 50 g (2 oz) hummus, sliced tomatoes, lettuce; 150 g (5 oz) low-fat natural yogurt with one piece of fruit, cup of tea.

Supper
Salade Niçoise (see recipe, page 76), wholemeal bread, two-fruit salad, 1 tbsp low-fat natural yogurt.

DAY EIGHTEEN

Breakfast
Either as Day 15 or Day 16.

Lunch
150 g (5 oz) cottage cheese mixed with chopped olives, radishes, spring onions, green salad, one piece wholemeal bread (with low-fat spread from daily allowance), apple, cup of tea.

Supper
Spaghetti with broccoli (see recipe, page 74), baked pepper salad (see recipe, page 77), banana split (1 tbsp iced yogurt instead of ice cream).

DAY NINETEEN

Breakfast
As Day 15.

Lunch
1 hard-boiled egg, 25 g (1 oz) feta cheese chopped into large mixed salad (from permitted vegetables), creamy low-cal dressing (see recipe, page 72), one piece of wholemeal bread toasted (with low-fat spread from daily allowance) as croutons, cup of tea.

Supper
Vegetable casserole (see recipe, page 73), 50 g (2 oz) rice (dried weight, preferably brown) boiled, salad of green pepper and medium onion chopped in rings, low-cal dressing (see recipe, page 72), one piece of fruit.

DAY TWENTY

Breakfast
Either as Day 15 or Day 16.

Lunch 150 g (5 oz) low-fat natural yogurt or 100 g (4 oz) fromage frais (8% fat), two pieces of fruit chopped in, sprinkling of sunflower seeds (optional).

Supper
100 g (4 oz) peeled prawns, large mixed salad, creamy low-cal dressing (see recipe, page 72), one slice of wholemeal bread, two-fruit salad, 1 tbsp frozen yogurt.

DAY TWENTY-ONE

Breakfast
Either as Day 15 or Day 16.

Lunch
Baked potato, 110 g (4 oz) baked beans, large green salad, low-cal dressing (see recipe, page 72), one piece of fruit, cup of tea.

Supper
150 g (5 oz) white fish baked, steamed or grilled, two tomatoes and one medium onion, sliced onto lettuce, low-cal dressing (see recipe, page 72), small bunch of grapes.

Your exercise programme

Increase the number of times you repeat each floor exercise by one, but with the Thigh Shaper, try a variation. Follow all the directions given in Week One but do it with your knees together, back as straight as ever (no leaning forward) and all your weight taken on the balls of your feet. Do ten 15cm (6in) rises, as before.

EXERCISE REPETITIONS: WEEK THREE	
Waist Twister	3
Hip and Thigh Toner	4
Thigh Shaper (variation)	10

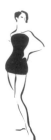

WEEK FOUR
Positive action: start at the top

JUST AS clothes with curve suit an Hourglass-type woman best, so do soft, wavy and not too severely short hairstyles. Actually, Hourglass women will often become very attached to their long wavy hair. Unless you're Jilly Cooper and your hair has become part of your image, it's more flattering if you don't wear it longer than your shoulders if you're older than thirty. For business, you will look more credible with a well-cut, mid-length style. If you really cannot bear to cut it, however, pin it up in an informal pleat or knot, tidy at the back and soft around your face.

Whatever length you favour, treat yourself to a good cut with a hair stylist who will take into consideration the weight and wave of your own hair and the shape of your face.

If you want to change the colour of your hair, bear in mind that its natural tone is the one which suits your skin and eye colour best. Unless you are aiming for a dramatic look (dark-haired Madonna was never meant to be a blonde), keep within your natural colour range. Dramatic changes can look sensational when you're young (and can afford an expensive professional style and its maintenance), but they are harsh and ageing to older skins.

Professionally done high- and low-lights can be a most flattering way of adding zing to your hair without clashing with the rest of your colouring. But it can be expensive. I would always say that if you had to choose, a good cut is the priority. Your own hair colour, glossy and healthy on this diet, will then look as exciting as can be.

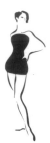

WEEK FOUR
Your diet

You are over the danger period of that third week. Although you may be disappointed that the scales do not register quite as much loss as you hoped I'm sure that by now you are feeling so much better—both slimmer and fitter—that you are quite happy to enter your fourth week. If Week Three had marked a plateau in your weight loss, then by the end of this fourth week I am pretty certain you will find you have lost more than you hoped.

It is so important to realize that even if you have a bad day when you do not manage to stick to your diet and the idea of doing any exercise other than from the sofa to the fridge seems anathema to you, it is not the beginning of the end. Just pick yourself up as quickly as possible and carry on where you left off and your weight will continue downwards.

DAY TWENTY-TWO
Breakfast
Half grapefruit (or other fruit from permitted list), 25 g (1 oz) muesli, bran flakes, puffed wheat, or other non-sweetened cereals (with skimmed milk from daily allowance), cup of tea or coffee.
Lunch
Tabbouleh (see recipe, page 77) in wholemeal pitta bread, grated carrot salad with orange juice as dressing, small bunch of grapes, cup of tea.
Supper
Mushroom omelette (see recipe, page 76), green beans and broccoli, or any two vegetables from permitted list, 150 g (5 oz) low-fat fruit yogurt.

DAY TWENTY-THREE
Breakfast
One egg poached, boiled or scrambled, one piece of toast (with low-fat spread from daily allowance), cup of tea or coffee.
Lunch
100 g (4 oz) cottage cheese with apple and orange chopped in, one piece of wholemeal bread, cup of tea.
Supper
Ratatouille (see recipe, page 74), with 50 g

(2 oz) rice (dried weight, preferably brown) boiled, one piece wholemeal bread, ginger bananas (see recipe, page 79).

DAY TWENTY-FOUR
Breakfast
Either as Day 22 or Day 23.
Lunch
Baked potato with low-cal coleslaw or homemade with creamy low-cal dressing (see recipe, page 72), 150 g (5 oz) low-fat fruit yogurt, cup of tea.
Supper
175 g (6 oz) chicken breast, rubbed with 1 tsp olive oil and herbs, grilled, selection of vegetables from permitted list, baked apple with 1 tsp honey and 1 tbsp low-fat natural yogurt.

DAY TWENTY-FIVE
Breakfast
Either as Day 22 or Day 23.
Lunch
300 ml (½ pt) any non-creamy packet soup or homemade vegetable soup (see recipe, page 75), one piece wholemeal bread/toast, banana, cup of tea.
Supper
175 g (6 oz) fresh (grilled) or tinned tuna (in brine not oil), large mixed salad, low-cal dressing (see recipe, page 72), fresh fruit salad (from permitted list), 1 tbsp low-fat natural yogurt.

DAY TWENTY-SIX
Breakfast
Either as Day 22 or Day 23.
Lunch
100 g (4 oz) cottage cheese, baked pepper salad (see recipe, page 77), one piece wholemeal bread or roll, one piece of fruit, cup of tea.
Supper
Seafood pasta (see recipe, page 74), green salad, low-cal dressing (see recipe, page 72), one piece of fruit.

HOURGLASS

Celebration treat:
buy something RED

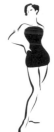

You've got there. Four weeks of a new way of eating and an exercise programme both of which are tailor-made for your body type and I hope you are really feeling more energetic, more attractive, more *you*. To celebrate, I would like to suggest that you go and buy yourself something red. It can be anything from a red scarf or handkerchief to red earrings, a jersey or—if you're feeling really triumphant—a red dress.

But remember, there are many shades of red. There are blue reds and orange reds; clear bright reds or muted, blended reds; light or deep reds. Before buying yourself your red treat, hold it under your chin to check it is a flattering red for you. The right red will give you a healthy glow, and your skin, hair and eyes will look more vibrant. The wrong red will make you pale and washed out. Any blemishes and dark shadows on your face are emphasized by the wrong colours.

Red is a marvellous colour. It lifts the spirits. It makes a definite statement; not 'poor little over-weight mousy me, please let me pass by unseen in the crowd', but rather , 'I AM FULL OF LIFE! I AM CONFIDENT, I AM HAPPY, LOOK AT ME!'

DAY TWENTY-SEVEN

Breakfast
Either as Day 22 or Day 23.

Lunch
Baked pepper and anchovy (see recipe, page 77), one wholemeal pitta bread, 150 g (5 oz) low-fat fruit yogurt, cup of tea.

Supper
Quarter of chicken, grilled or dry roasted, broccoli, green beans (or other permitted vegetables) steamed or boiled, two-fruit salad with 1 tbsp low-fat yogurt (or frozen yogurt).

DAY TWENTY-EIGHT

Breakfast
Either as Day 22 or day 23.

Lunch
Three fruits from permitted list made into fruit salad with 100 g (4 oz) low-fat natural yogurt, 1 tbsp muesli stirred in, cup of tea.

Supper
Chick pea curry (see recipe, page 74), 25 g (1 oz) rice (dried weight, preferably brown) boiled, large green salad, low-cal dressing (see recipe, page 72), one piece of fruit.

Your exercise programme

Increase your exercises by one and continue with the Thigh Shaper as outlined in the box below. You should be feeling so good by now and there will be a real improvement in your shape. I hope that your exercise programme will have become second nature to you. But even if you have lazy lapses, or occasional food binges, don't give up in disgust. Exercise is wonderful as an anti-depressant. If you find yourself in a low mood, rather than slumping in front of the telly or dashing for the fridge, try doing something which raises your heart rate like digging the garden, playing tennis, taking a brisk walk around the park. I guarantee that after any of these activities you will have forgotten that depressed, sluggish feeling. In addition to the exercise programme included here, I hope that from your exercise tapes or classes you have found other spot exercises to add variety and enjoyment.

EXERCISE REPETITIONS: WEEK FOUR	
Waist Twister	4
Hip and Thigh Toner	5
Thigh Shaper (variation)	15

RECIPE SUPPLEMENT

Low-Cal Dressing

(Make up a jar and use on salads when necessary: 1 dessertsp = 40 calories)

3 tbsp good olive oil
3 tbsp water
3 tbsp wine or cider vinegar
1 clove garlic, crushed
½ tsp salt
1 tsp dried tarragon

1 Put all the ingredients into a screw top jar and shake. Let stand a few hours before using.
2 To vary, use different herbs, or leave out garlic and add 1 tsp capers, liquidise the dressing in a blender. Or add 1 tsp Dijon mustard and 3 tsp apple juice instead of water.

Stir-Fry Chicken and Vegetables

(Serves 1)

25 g (1 oz) brown rice
1 tsp low-fat spread from daily allowance
100 g (4 oz) chicken breast, skinned and sliced coarsely
1 Spanish onion, sliced finely
3 sticks celery, sliced
75 g (3 oz) mushrooms, sliced
225 g (8 oz) bean sprouts (fresh or tinned)
2 carrots, coarsely grated
soy sauce/tamari to taste

1 Cook rice in boiling water.
2 In heavy frying pan or wok melt low-fat spread, fry chicken slices until they begin to change colour.
3 Add the prepared vegetables, onion first, then celery, mushrooms, and lastly bean sprouts and carrot.

4 Add splash of soy sauce/tamari to taste. Serve on drained rice.

Creamy Low-Cal Dressing

(Make up a jar and use when necessary: 1 dessertsp = 10 calories)

100 g (4 oz) low-fat cottage cheese
100 g (4 oz) low-fat natural yogurt
½ green pepper, chopped
4 sliced radishes
2 dessertsp chives
1 dessertsp poppy seeds
salt, pepper and pinch basil/oregano to taste

1 Put all ingredients into a blender or food processor. Keep in a jar and use on coleslaw, mixed salads, or in baked potatoes.

Tofu Stir-Fry

(Serves 1)

50 g (2 oz) brown rice
110 g (4 oz) tofu
1 tsp vegetable oil
1 tsp tamari/soy sauce
1 stalk celery, sliced
wedge of white cabbage, coarsely shredded
110 g (4 oz) bean sprouts
25 g (1 oz) water chestnuts (optional)
2 tsp cornflour
1 tsp water
2 tsp tamari/soy sauce

1 Put rice on to boil.
2 Cut tofu into bite-sized pieces.
3 Heat oil in frying pan. Put tofu in pan, sprinkle with tamari/soy sauce. Carefully brown the tofu sides and put aside.

4 Add celery and cabbage to pan, stir-fry 3 minutes. Add bean sprouts and water chestnuts, stir-fry for another 3 minutes.
5 Mix cornflour with water and tamari/soy sauce. Pour mixture over vegetables and stir well. Add tofu, mix gently and cover.
6 Steam for a few minutes until sauce is thickened.
7 Serve with boiled, drained rice.

Cheese-Baked Cauliflower

(Serves 1)

half large head cauliflower
1 egg
1 tbsp skimmed milk
generous pinch dill
25 g (1 oz) cheddar/emmenthal, grated
1 tbsp curd/low-fat soft cheese
salt, pepper

1 Heat oven to 190°C (375°F, gas mark 5)
2 Break cauliflower head into florets, steam or boil in minimum amount of water until just soft.
3 Beat together egg, milk, dill, cheeses, and season.
4 Put cooked cauliflower in small casserole dish, pour on cheesy mixture, cover with lid or foil and cook for about 10 minutes, when egg will have begun to set and cheese to melt.

Stir-Fry Vegetables and Rice

(Serves 1)

50 g (2 oz) brown rice
2 tsp sesame/vegetable oil
1 clove garlic, chopped fine
pinch ginger (1 tsp fresh grated)
selection of vegetables from permitted list (chopped finely, to fill 450 ml [16 fl oz] measuring jug)
25 g (1 oz) cheddar cheese, grated
tamari/soy sauce

1 Put rice on to boil.
2 Heat oil in large frying pan, add garlic and ginger, then add vegetables needing most cooking, ie carrots and any other root vegetables.
3 Stir constantly, adding the vegetables that need

less cooking as you go along, ie spring onions, green peppers, mushrooms, bean sprouts. Add a little water if necessary to prevent sticking. Cook until tender/crisp.
4 Serve cooked rice with vegetables, sprinkle cheese on top and add tamari/soy sauce to taste.

Stuffed Tomatoes

(Serves 1)

3 medium sized tomatoes
½ cup cooked rice (brown)
2 pecan nuts, broken
50 g (2 oz) low-fat (curd) cheese
2 tbsp chives/spring onions
pinch dried basil
salt, pepper

1 Cut a 'lid' off the top of each tomato, scoop out and chop pulp.
2 Leave tomato shells upside down on kitchen paper to drain.
3 Add cooked rice, nuts, curd cheese, onion and basil to tomato pulp and beat well. Season to taste.
4 Fill tomatoes with stuffing mixture, replace lids, leave to stand a little before serving.

Vegetable Casserole

(Serves 1)

450 g (1 lb) selection of vegetables from permitted list, eg courgettes, mushrooms, broccoli, carrots, peppers, Brussels sprouts

300 ml (½ pt) water
100 g (4 oz) lentils (dry weight)
1 clove garlic, chopped
1 tsp paprika
salt, pepper
1 vegetable stock cube

1 Chop vegetables, not too small, and put in a small casserole with water, lentils, garlic and paprika. Add salt and pepper and crumbled stock cube and cover with lid.
2 Put in moderate oven—180°C (350°F, gas mark 4)—and cook for about 1 hour, or until tender.

Chick Pea Curry

(Serves 1)

75 g (3 oz) dried chick peas soaked overnight
  (or 215 g [7 oz] tinned)
1 small onion, chopped fine
1–2 cloves garlic, chopped fine
2.5cms (1in) fresh ginger root, grated
1 fresh green chilli, finely chopped (optional)
1–2 tsp curry powder (to taste)
2 large, chopped tomatoes, or 215 g (7 oz) tinned
juice of half lemon
salt, pepper
1 tbsp low-fat natural yogurt

1 If using dried and soaked chick peas, cook in water for an hour or so until tender. Drain cooked or tinned chick peas.
2 In heavy frying pan melt 1 tsp of low-fat margarine from allowance and add onion, garlic, ginger and chilli. Fry gently for 3–4 minutes until soft and browning.
3 Stir in curry powder and cook for another 2 minutes. Add chopped tomatoes and lemon juice.
4 Add chick peas. Stir and simmer 10–15 minutes. Add a little water if curry starts to dry out.
5 Season with salt and pepper, take off heat, stir in yogurt and serve.

Ratatouille

(Serves 1)

225 g (8 oz) courgettes
1 large aubergine
1 green pepper
400 g (15 oz) tin of tomatoes
2 bay leaves
1 large onion, chopped
2 cloves garlic, chopped
salt, pepper

1 Slice the courgettes and aubergine. Core and seed pepper and cut into strips.
2 Place tomatoes in a large saucepan and add the rest of the ingredients.
3 Bring to the boil and simmer for 20 minutes or until vegetables are tender, skim off any sediment. If too much liquid remains, raise heat and boil more vigorously, without the lid, until sauce is thickened.

Seafood Pasta

(Serves 1)

50 g (2 oz) pasta
½ clove garlic, chopped
juice and grated skin ½ lime
75 g (3 oz) prawns
1 tbsp fresh dill (1 tbsp dried)
2 tbsp low-fat natural yogurt
1 tbsp skimmed milk
salt, pepper
2 tsp grated parmesan cheese

1 Cook pasta in boiling water, until tender but *al dente*.
2 Meanwhile put garlic and lime juice and grated skin in small pan and cook gently.
3 When the pasta is nearly ready, add prawns and dill to garlic and lime mixture and heat thoroughly, but don't overcook.
4 Whisk together yogurt and milk and add to the mixture. Heat thoroughly, *but do not boil*. Season to taste.
5 Drain pasta, pour sauce over and sprinkle on parmesan.

Spaghetti with Broccoli

(Serves 1)

1 clove garlic, chopped fine
1 tsp of low-fat spread from daily allowance
175 g (6 oz) broccoli
4–5 tbsp water
50 g (2 oz) spaghetti or other pasta
salt, pepper
2 tsp grated parmesan cheese

1 Gently fry garlic in low-fat spread for 1–2 minutes.
2 Dice broccoli and add to garlic in pan, stir for 2 minutes. Add water, cover and simmer for 10 minutes until broccoli stem is softening. If pan is dry, add a little more water.
3 Cook pasta in pan of lightly salted boiling water for about 7–8 minutes until al dente.
4 Drain pasta and toss with broccoli (which should have a little garlicky juice). Season with salt and milled pepper to taste and sprinkle parmesan on top.

Vegetable Soup

(4 Servings)

1 medium size onion
1 medium size potato
1 medium size parsnip
100 g (4 oz) carrots
25 g (1 oz) low-fat spread from daily allowance
2 tbsp chopped parsley
½ tsp mixed herbs
nutmeg to taste
1.2 l (2 pt) vegetable stock (or 2 cubes)
1 small leek
50 g (2 oz) cabbage
salt, pepper

1 Chop onion, potato, parsnip and carrots. Melt half the low-fat spread in a saucepan and sauté the vegetables gently stirring occasionally, until the onion is transparent.
2 Add parsley, herbs, nutmeg and stock and bring to the boil. Cover and simmer for 30 minutes.
3 Cool a little and then liquidise in blender.
4 Meanwhile, finely shred the leek and cabbage and sauté them in the remaining low-fat spread until just softening. Add to blended soup, simmer gently for 10 minutes. Adjust seasoning.

Kyoto Trout Salad

(Serves 1)

1 medium size trout, skinned and filleted
juice of 2 lemons
1 carrot
5-cm (2-in) piece of cucumber
handful of lambs' tongue lettuce (or rocket/frisée)
¼ avocado, sliced
¼ red pepper, cut in strips
¼ green pepper, cut in strips
1 tsp olive oil

1 Put trout fillets into a shallow bowl and pour over lemon juice. Leave all day, or overnight to marinade, turning occasionally.
2 Drain fillets from lemon juice and cut into chunks.
3 Cut carrot and cucumber lengthwise, into fine sticks, and mix with the lambs' tongue lettuce, avocado slices and red and green pepper. Add the trout pieces.
4 Arrange on your plate and trickle the olive oil over the mixture.

Bean and Lentil Salad

(Serves 1)

75 g (3 oz) (cooked weight) cooked or tinned kidney beans
25 g (1 oz) (cooked weight) green lentils
¼ red pepper, cut in strips
¼ green pepper, cut in strips
¼ spanish onion, cut in fine rings
1 tsp lemon juice
1 tsp olive oil
salt, pepper
handful of chopped parsley and/or chives

1 Put the beans, lentils, peppers and onion rings in a bowl.
2 Pour on the lemon juice and the oil and mix well. Season and toss the parsley and or chives on top.

Stir-Fry Beef with Mange-Tout

(Serves 1)

75 g (3 oz) beef fillet, cut across grain into thin strips
soy sauce
1 tsp vegetable (or sesame) oil
75 g (3 oz) mange-tout, topped and tailed
dash of sherry

1 Sprinkle beef strips with soy sauce and leave for at least an hour.
2 Preheat wok or heavy frying pan with 1 tsp oil.
3 Stir-fry beef strips for 2 minutes. Add prepared mange-tout and continue to stir.
4 After another 2 minutes, or when cooked, pour in a teaspoon of soy sauce and a dash of sherry. Mix all ingredients together for another minute and serve.

Tandoori Chicken

(Serves 1)

1 tsp Tandoori Masala barbecue powder
1 clove garlic, minced or crushed
1 dessertsp tomato purée
1 tbsp natural low-fat yogurt
¼ chicken portion

1 Mix all the spices and tomato purée into yogurt.
2 Cut long slices in the chicken flesh and cover with the yogurt mixture, working it into the flesh. Leave for as long as possible, preferably all day or overnight.
3 Scrape off any excess mixture and grill for 15 minutes each side, or until properly cooked (stick a skewer into the thickest part and make sure the juices are no longer pink).

Quick Pea Soup

(Serves 1)

100 g (4 oz) frozen peas
300 ml (½ pt) chicken OR vegetable stock (or ½ cube)
½–1 tbsp fresh mint (optional)
1 tbsp fromage frais 8% OR natural yogurt
salt, pepper

1 Simmer peas in stock for 2–3 minutes, or until cooked. Add chopped mint, if using.
2 Liquidize the soup with the fromage frais or yogurt.
3 Re-heat gently if you need to, but *do not boil*. Season to taste.

Mushroom Omelette

(Serves 1)

1 tsp low-fat spread from daily allowance
100 g (4 oz) sliced mushrooms
2 eggs
1 tbsp fromage frais 8% OR natural yogurt
salt, pepper
fresh parsley or other herbs

1 In small heavy frying pan melt the low-fat spread and add the mushrooms.
2 Cook gently until browning. Remove from pan.

3 Beat eggs with fromage frais or yogurt, add seasoning and pour mixture into pan.
4 With wooden spoon, draw in the setting edges towards the centre. When set, but still quite moist, arrange mushrooms and parsley on one half of pan and fold other half of omelette over.
5 Serve on warm plate.

Spanish Omelette

(Serves 1)

1 tsp low-fat spread from daily allowance
100 g (4 oz) prepared vegetables, eg sliced courgettes, red pepper, mushrooms, peas, fine chopped carrot
1 dessertsp chopped parsley
salt, pepper
2 eggs

1 Heat the fat in a small heavy-bottomed frying pan.
2 Add the mixed vegetables and stir until they begin to soften, turn heat low and cook until *al dente*, stirring frequently.
3 Add chopped parsley, salt and pepper.
4 Lightly beat eggs, season lightly and pour mixture onto vegetables in pan.
5 Stir gently with a fork until eggs begin to set. Serve from pan.

Salade Niçoise

(Serves 1)

lettuce leaves
100 g (4 oz) cooked green beans, cooled
2 tomatoes, sliced
100 g (4 oz) tuna in brine
1 hard boiled egg, quartered
4 anchovy fillets, drained
4 black olives
1 dessertsp low-cal dressing (see page 72)
salt, pepper

1 Arrange a bed of lettuce leaves, add the beans and sliced tomatoes.
2 Pile the drained and flaked tuna in the middle and arrange the egg quarters around the edge.
3 Garnish with the anchovies and black olives. Sprinkle on the dressing and season to taste.

Red Cabbage, Apple and Hazelnut Salad

(Serves 1)

175 g (6 oz) red cabbage
1 eating apple (cox/russet)
25 g (1 oz) raisins
1 dessertsp low-cal dressing (see page 72)
25 g (1 oz) hazelnuts

1 Wash and shred cabbage finely. Core and chop apple coarsely.
2 Combine cabbage, apple and raisins in a bowl, pour on dressing and mix well. Ideally leave for about 2 hours before eating.
3 Sprinkle on chopped hazelnuts just before serving.

Tabbouleh

(Serves 1)

This dish traditionally comes loaded with olive oil but this is a recipe for a much less oil-rich (and therefore less calorie-rich) version.

40 g (1½ oz) bulgar/cracked wheat
4–6 spring onions, finely chopped
2 tbsp fresh parsley, finely chopped
1 tbsp fresh mint
7.5-cms (3-in) piece of cucumber
1–2 tomatoes, chopped
juice of ½ lemon
1 dessertsp low-cal dressing (see above)
salt, pepper

1 Pour boiling water over the wheat and leave for 10 minutes to swell. Drain in a sieve and with your hands squeeze out as much excess water as possible.
2 Put wheat in a bowl and add chopped onions, parsley, mint, cucumber and tomatoes (minus their seeds and watery pulp).
3 Mix in lemon juice, low-cal dressing, salt and pepper to taste.
4 If possible, allow to stand for a while to let flavours blend.

Baked Pepper Salad

(Serves 1)

2 red firm fresh peppers
1 dessertsp low-cal dressing (see above)
fresh parsley (optional)

1 Heat up grill. Place whole red pepper under grill and cook each side until the flesh is charred and blistering.
2 When all sides have blistered and peppers have cooled enough to touch, run under cold water and peel off outer, burnt skin.
3 Slice in half, de-seed and de-core, and slice flesh lengthways into strips.
4 Place on side-plate and dribble low-cal dressing over strips. Serve with chopped fresh parsley if available.

Baked Pepper & Anchovy

(Serves 1)

1 fresh red pepper
2 anchovy fillets, drained
2 cloves garlic, sliced fine
1 tomato sliced into four
1 tsp good olive oil

1 Set oven to moderately high 190°C (375°F, gas mark 5).
2 Quarter red pepper, de-core and de-seed, and place skin side down in small ovenproof dish.
3 In each quarter place half anchovy fillet, 3 slices of garlic and slice of tomato.
4 Brush each quarter with olive oil.
5 Cook in oven for 30–40 minutes. Serve hot or cold.

Crudités with Crab Dip

(Serves 2)

175 g (6 oz) can of crabmeat
150 g (5 oz) low-fat natural yogurt
1 tsp lemon juice
salt, pepper
2 carrots
1.3 cm (½ in) cucumber
2 sticks of celery
1 red/green pepper

1 Drain brine off crabmeat and mix with yogurt and lemon juice. Season with salt and pepper to taste.
2 Wash and slice carrots, cucumber and celery into strips.
3 Halve red/green pepper, de-seed and cut into strips.
4 Put crab dip into a small bowl and arrange vegetables on a plate.

Mushroom and Pepper Risotto

(Serves 1)

1 clove garlic, minced or finely chopped
½ medium onion, chopped
1 tsp olive oil
175 g (6 oz) mushrooms (ideally large, field
    mushrooms), diced
½ green/red pepper, de-seeded and diced
50 g (2 oz) white round grain rice (preferably risotto
    rice, but pudding rice will do)
1 vegetable stock cube
1 dessertsp sherry (optional)
handful of parsley, chopped
4 spring onions, chopped (optional)

1 Gently fry the garlic and onion in oil in a heavy, medium-sized frying pan, until transparent.
2 Add mushrooms and diced pepper and stir for a minute or so, then add rice and continue stirring.
3 Make 300 ml (½ pt) of vegetable stock with cube and add this to the rice and vegetable mixture. Add sherry, if using it.
4 Simmer gently in the uncovered pan for 25–30 minutes until the rice is cooked. If the mixture dries out before the rice is properly cooked, add a little more water.
5 Sprinkle the parsley and optional spring onions on top and serve.

Fish Florentine

(Serves 1)

175 g (6 oz) fillet of white fish
120 g (4 oz) frozen chopped spinach, thawed
25 g (1 oz) parmesan or cheddar cheese, grated
pepper

1 Place fillet in bottom of small, shallow baking dish.
2 Having squeezed all excess moisture out of the spinach, place over fish.
3 Sprinkle with cheese and season with pepper.
4 Bake in hot oven, 200°C (400°F, gas mark 6) for 20 minutes.

Crunchy Chicken Salad

(Serves 1)

1 chicken breast
1 carrot, diced
1 tbsp low-fat natural yogurt
1 tsp calorie-reduced mayonnaise
1 small clove garlic, chopped small
pinch paprika
salt, pepper
4 spring onions, sliced
½ eating apple, cored and cubed
½ bunch watercress, minus stalks
2 tbsp shredded red or hard white cabbage
½ red pepper, de-seeded and sliced

1 Put chicken breast in small pan, cover with water and simmer for 25 minutes, remove skin and add carrots. Cook for another 5 minutes, until chicken is cooked and carrots still firm..
2 Drain and cool. Cut chicken flesh into strips.
3 Mix yogurt and mayonnaise and add garlic, paprika, salt and pepper to taste.
4 Mix chicken strips with carrots, spring onions, apple, watercress leaves, hard cabbage, red pepper. Add dressing mixture. Toss and chill in fridge before serving.

Papaya and Mango Fruit Salad

(Serves 2)

1 ripe papaya
1 ripe mango
rind and juice of ½ lime

1 Peel, halve and de-seed papaya, slice lengthwise and then cut into cubes.
2 Peel mango and slice flesh off stone, cut into cubes.
4 Mix fruit together in a bowl with finely grated zest and juice of half a lime.
5 Divide into two servings.

Orange Sorbet

(Serves 1)

1 dessertsp lemon juice
1 tsp liquid honey
grated rind of ½ orange
half 175 g (8 oz) can unsweetened orange juice
1 small egg white
slices of orange to garnish

1 Mix lemon juice with honey and make it up to 150 ml (¼ pint) with warm water.
2 Add orange rind and juice and pour mixture into a 600 ml (1 pint) bowl and put in freezer.
3 When half frozen, mash with a fork into a semi-frozen pulp.
4 Whisk egg white until stiff and fold into the mixture with a metal spoon.
5 Return to freezer and freeze until firm.
6 Before serving, leave it in the refrigerator for 15–20 minutes to soften it slightly. Serve with an orange twist.

Rhubarb Fool

(Serves 1)

175 g (6 oz) rhubarb
1 lemon
liquid sweetener
150 g (5 oz) low-fat natural yogurt

1 Top and tail the rhubarb, then wash and cut into chunks.
2 Put rhubarb into a small saucepan with 1 tbsp lemon juice, ½ tsp lemon zest and 1 tbsp water. Simmer gently.
3 When cooked, add liquid sweetener to taste.
4 Put aside to cool. Then blend mixture in a liquidizer.
5 Pour rhubarb into a bowl and fold in the yogurt. Chill and serve.

Ginger Bananas

(Serves 1)

1 ripe banana
1 piece of crystallized ginger, chopped
few almond flakes
1 tbsp fromage frais 8%/frozen yogurt

1 Slice banana into pudding bowl.
2 Sprinkle ginger over bananas, top with almonds and serve with fromage frais or frozen yogurt.

6 WEEKS LATER 8

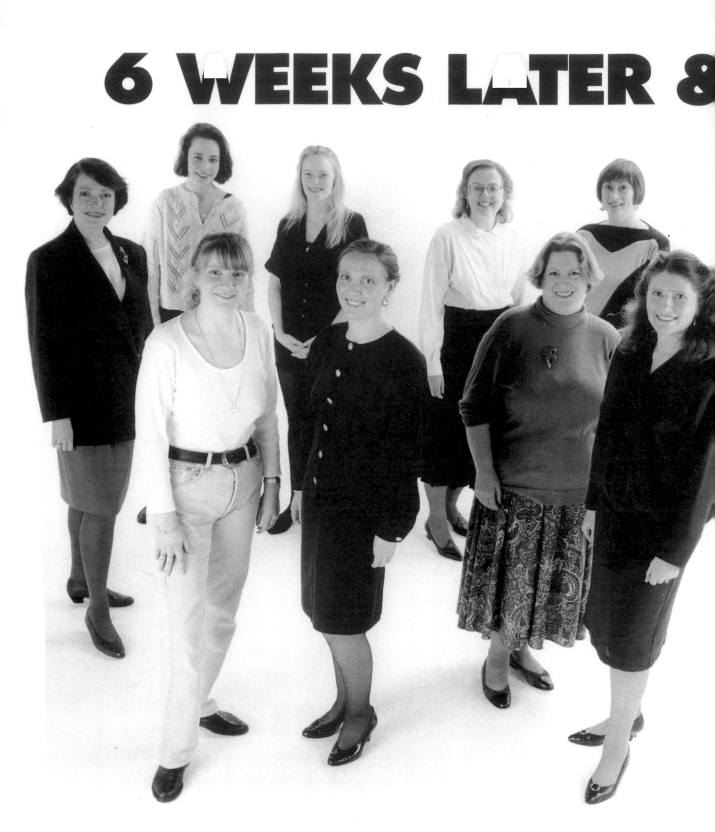

Here are some of our volunteer dieters six weeks later. Some have gone on since to lose even more than they did in the six-week trial.

SO MUCH LIGHTER

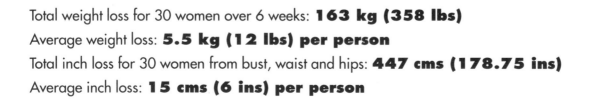

Total weight loss for 30 women over 6 weeks: **163 kg (358 lbs)**

Average weight loss: **5.5 kg (12 lbs) per person**

Total inch loss for 30 women from bust, waist and hips: **447 cms (178.75 ins)**

Average inch loss: **15 cms (6 ins) per person**

THE BODY BREAKTHROUGH

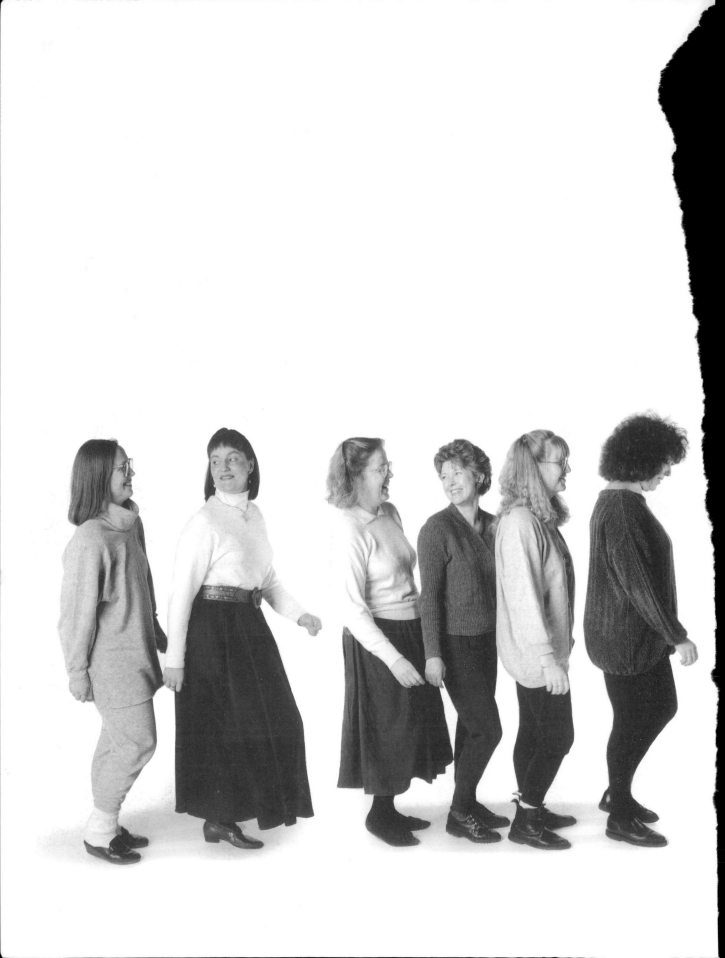

THE
BODY
BREAKTHROUGH

BEL HISLOP

DISCOVER WHICH BODY SHAPE YOU ARE AND
UNLOCK THE KEY TO DRAMATIC WEIGHT LOSS

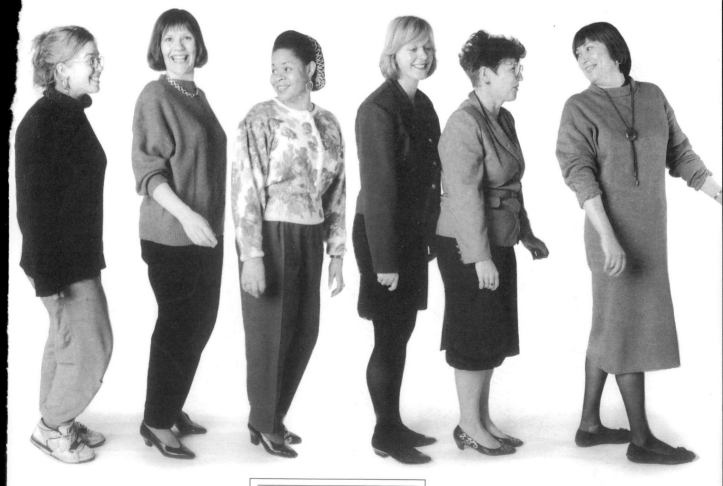

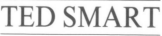

TED SMART

Acknowledgements

The author and publisher would like to thank all the friends, and clients who became friends, for volunteering to be guinea pig dieters and making the whole thing such a success and such fun to do. Their comments and experiences helped clarify and refine the diet and exercise programmes and we are very grateful for their hard work, enthusiasm, good will AND SUCCESS.

Thanks to my associate Liz Thesen for administrative help and support and for being so useful in discussions about Triangle-type style, dieting and exercise.

Grateful thanks too to Carrick James and John Goodwin of Carrick James Market Research for invaluable help and advice in formulating and computing the questionnaire.

I would like to thank photographers Helen Pask and Jon Stewart for their patience and sensitivity during the photographic sessions, and Susan Greenhill for her sense of humour and skill in making me look as much like I'd like to look as possible.

I would also like to thank Heath at Pineapple Press Office, Ellen King at Freed's, and BHS for loan of leotards and tights, and for their efficiency and helpfulness in all their dealings.

Particular thanks to Emma Callery, the book's editor, for her immediate enthusiasm and sympathy for the message of *Body Breakthrough*, and for all her hard work in bringing it to press. Many thanks too to Denise Bates, Editor and overseer, and to the dynamic publicity team of Niccy Cowen and Sarah Bennie. Of course, particular thanks to my agent Deborah Rogers and publisher Amelia Thorpe; I am grateful for their continual enthusiasm and support.

I would also like to thank Random House's supremo Gail Rebuck who, in her hectic round, still managed to read the synopsis and make the inspired suggestion that it should be a reversible book, with two interlinked jackets.

My warmest thanks to my family, Michael, Sam and Marthe, for their continual help, support and understanding while I have been preoccupied with women and their different body types.

Most special thanks to Ben and Lily Dunn and to Nick Ostler for their generous good humour, various help and comments, and particularly for the support of my friend and collaborator, Jane Dunn.

For further information on personal and corporate consultations
on image and diet, contact:
WORKING IMAGE, PO Box 3000, London N5 1WW, England

CONTENTS

DISCOVER YOUR

Every woman falls into one of four body-type categories. The type you are can have far-reaching significance in your life; what you eat, how you exercise, what you wear, how you age, what illnesses you are prone to, even how you feel. It is important to be able to identify what body type you are: do you recognise yourself in one of these shapes?

The questionnaire over the page will either reinforce your decision or hel exactly which body-type category you fall into.

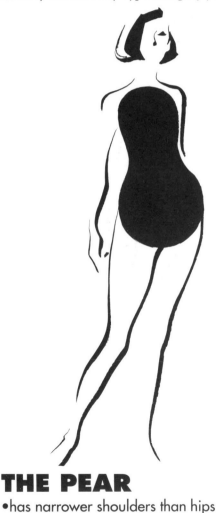

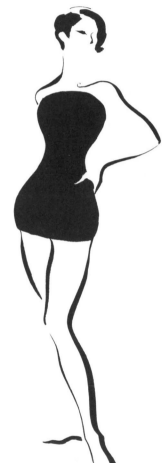

THE PEAR
•has narrower shoulders than hips
•has less fat above the waist than below
•always has a waist and flattish tummy
•has curvy hips and thighs.

THE HOURGLASS
•has balanced shoulders and hips
•has fat equally distributed on bust and hips
•retains a waist however heavy she gets
•always has a curve to her hips however thin
    she gets.

BODY TYPE

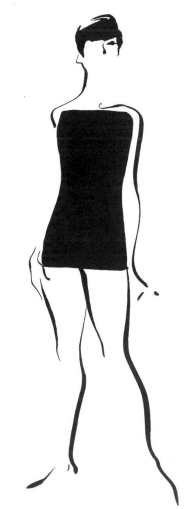

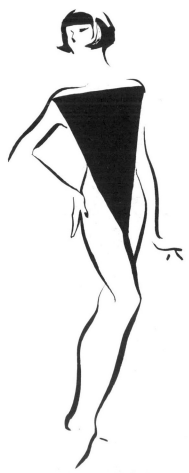

THE RECTANGLE

- has balanced shoulders and hips
- has not got a sharply defined waist
- has a strong body often with slim legs
- has straight hips and a flattish bottom.

THE TRIANGLE

- has broader shoulders than hips
- has a waist and *straight* hips tapering to thighs
- has a narrow pelvis and flat bottom
- has lean lower legs.

QUESTIONNAIRE

For each question, please read alternatives carefully and tick one answer in the boxes at the right hand side

BODY SHAPE

1 Please look at yourself in a mirror, without your clothes, and face-on. Do you have a body shape with:

   a shoulder and hip of similar width, with little or no waist? [C]

   b shoulder and hip of similar width, with a defined waist? [B]

   c shoulders narrower than hips, with a slim waist? [A]

   d broader shoulders with tapering hips and a defined waist? [D]

2a Now look at yourself sideways. Is your bottom:

   a flat and tucked in? [C&D]

   b a more rounded curve? [A&B]

2b Still looking sideways, do you carry most weight:

   a in front of you on bust, tummy and spare tyre (roll of fat above waist)? [C&D]

   b behind you, on bottom? [A]

   c equally front and back, on bust and bottom? [B]

3 Now looking at yourself from the back, do you have noticeable 'saddlebags' (curvy deposits of fat on the outer thighs)?

   a No [C&D]

   b Yes [A&B]

4 With a tape measure, measure your waist and then the *biggest* part of your hips. Is your hip measurement:

   a MORE than 25 cms (10 ins) bigger than your waist? [A&B]

   b LESS than 25 cms (10 ins) bigger than your waist? [C&D]

WEIGHT DISTRIBUTION

5 Still looking at yourself in the mirror, face-on and then side-on.
When you put on weight is it more noticeable:

    a in your face-on body profile, *ie* you get *wider*?   [A&B]

    b in your side-on body profile, *ie* you get *deeper*?   [C&D]

6a When you are/were very slim and put on those *first* 3 kg (7 lbs)
of weight, where was it most noticeable:

    a *lower* hips and thighs, and a bit on tummy?   [B]

    b tummy and spare tyre?   [C]

    c *lower* hips and thighs?   [A]

    d tummy, upper chest and face?   [D]

6b When you are more than 3 kg (7 lbs) overweight, where does
your excess weight accumulate:

    a on tummy, upper chest, upper arms, *upper* hips, *ie* just below
waist, and inside thighs, BUT retaining a waist?   [D]

    b most on *lower* hips and thighs, little on top half of body?   [A]

    c pretty much all over, ie on bust and predominantly on hips,
BUT retaining a waist?   [B]

    d on tummy, spare tyre, bust, back and *upper* hips, losing what
little waist you might have had?   [C]

7 If you were to put on 3 kg (7 lbs) would you get noticeably fatter in the face?

    a Yes   [C&D]

    b No   [A&B]

8 If you were to put on 3 kg (7 lbs) would your hands and feet get
noticeably more fleshy?

    a Yes   [B&C]

    b No   [A&D]

ENERGY LEVELS AND EATING PATTERNS

9 Regardless of demands of work, children, etc, when naturally are you most *mentally* energetic?

    a slow to get going, most *creative* energy at night [C]

    b physical energy levels pretty constant all day, *creative* energy increases from afternoon into evening [A]

    c brightest in the morning, early to bed [D]

    d spurts and slumps of *creative* energy throughout the day [B]

10 Regardless of the social and work demands in your life (and when you're not on a diet), which best describes your natural eating habits:

    a like to snack through the day [B]

    b irregular or erratic meal times, no heavy meals at night [D]

    c healthy appetite—start eating can't stop [C]

    d can go for quite a long time without food, seldom binge [A]

EXERCISE

11 How sporty were you as a schoolgirl?

    a keen to get out of the gym periods and ferocious hockey matches – not at all competitive but happy to play tennis and rounders [A]

    b very sporty and enthusiastic, loved athletics, team sports, etc, likely to enter for as many events as possible on Sports Day [C]

    c sporty and very competitive, not so keen on team sports but good at individual athletic events, competitive tennis/squash/gymnastics and dancing [D]

    d pretty easy-going either way, good at team sports, not very competitive, more interested in the camaraderie [B]

12 **If you want to lose weight, do you:**

    a go on a diet and not worry about increasing your exercise?   [A]

    b go on a diet and *think* about doing more exercise but not be
       very enthusiastic about it?   [B]

    c go on a diet and work out a practical plan for doing more
       regular exercise—and intend to keep to it?   [C]

    d you're already doing quite a bit of exercise, so you go on a diet
       and increase your exercise even more?   [D]

13 When you're engaged in a vigorous programme of exercise and sport
    would you get depressed and put on weight if you gave it up?

    a Yes   [C&D]

    b No   [A&B]

Now add up all the capital letters in the boxes you have ticked.

A predominance of As and you're a **PEAR** type

A predominance of Bs and you're an **HOURGLASS** type

A predominance of Cs and you're a **RECTANGLE** type

A predominance of Ds and you're a **TRIANGLE** type

If you have no clear predominance of any one letter, then add up just the ticks from the *Body Shape* and *Weight Distribution* sections. They are more accurately indicative of your body type.

Finally, check your own physical characteristics against the checklist over the page which will help to clarify your type (but obviously not everyone will conform to *all* the characteristics of their type). The four body types, however, apply to all women, whatever their race or nationality.

If you have passed the menopause and your shape has thickened, particularly around the waist—a Triangle type, for example, can become more like a Rectangle—then answer the questions as if for your original shape and follow the appropriate body-type programme.

THE F UR BODY TY ES

These illustrations show you exactly where each body type is most likely to put on weight.

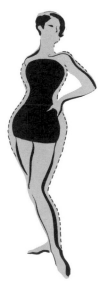

THE PEAR

has narrower shoulders than hips
has less fat above the waist than below
always has a waist and flattish tummy
has curvy hips and thighs
If you:
- put weight predominantly on your *lower* hips, bottom and thighs
- have a small bust in proportion to your hips
- have delicate shoulders and neck
- rarely put weight on your shoulders and face

then you are a Pear Type

For your complete four-week diet and exercise package: turn to page 25 *in the reverse section of the book*

THE HOURGLASS

has balanced shoulders and hips
has fat equally distributed on bust and hips
retains a waist, however heavy she gets
always has a curve to her hips however thin she gets
If you:
- put weight on all over, but particularly on *lower* hips and bottom
- have a rounded bosom and rounded bottom
- always keep your waist
- have basically *rounded* limbs

then you are an Hourglass Type

For your complete four-week diet and exercise package: turn to page 49 *in the reverse section of the book*

THE RECTANGLE

has balanced shoulders and hips

has *not* got a sharply defined waist, even when slim

has a strong and sturdy body often with slim legs

has straight hips and a flattish bottom

If you:

- have lean legs and a flattish bottom which gets fatter and squarer from the waist down
- put weight on torso, predominantly on stomach, spare tyre, breasts, upper back and upper hips
- lose what little waist you have when overweight (become more of a 'cube' than a Rectangle)
- become *deeper*, ie put weight on the front
- have basically *straight* limbs

then you are a Rectangle Type

For your complete four-week diet and exercise package: turn to page 25

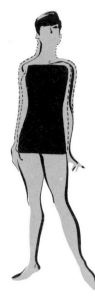

THE TRIANGLE

has broader shoulders than hips

has a waist and *straight* hips which taper towards thighs

has a narrow pelvis and a flat bottom

has lean lower legs

If you:

- look top heavy when you put on weight
- put weight on predominantly above the hip bone; on tummy, chest, face, spare tyre, upper arms, *upper* hips and *inner* thighs
- have straight hips which get boxy when overweight
- get fleshy and squarer in the back and chest when overweight

then you are a Triangle Type

For your complete four-week diet and exercise package: turn to page 49

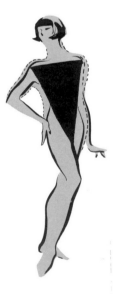

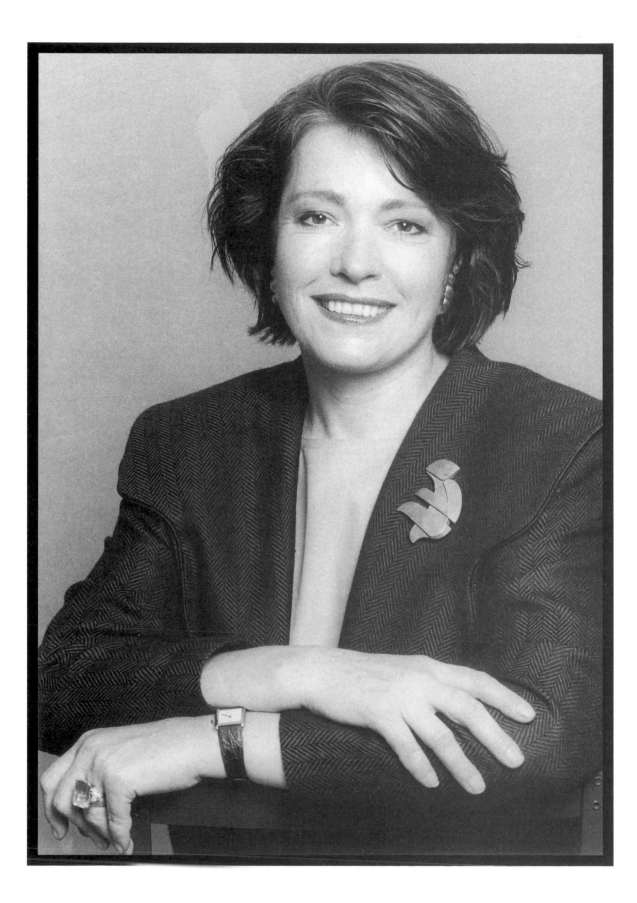

INTRODUCTION

I AM a style and personal development consultant and after years of work and discussion with thousands of women clients and reading of scientific papers, I have discovered a simple truth about women's body shapes—we are not all the same physical type and do not share the same basic shape. Furthermore, our different body shapes indicate different metabolisms and different dietary and exercise needs.

I have always known that I was a different basic shape from my two sisters because what I wore didn't necessarily suit them and vice versa. We also put weight on in different areas and in different proportions. We cannot change this basic underlying shape although we can refine features of it through diet and exercise. But only when I began my training as a style consultant did I realize how important and unchanging these different body shapes are. Which body shape you are is significant in many ways, most noticeably in the way your body responds to food and exercise.

This simple fact, that we have different shapes and therefore different metabolisms, is the basis of this book—a breakthrough among diet books. It is backed up by some really remarkable scientific evidence (see below) which has shown that the differences in female body shape and where fat is deposited indicate something of central importance to everyone wishing to understand themselves and their bodies.

This central idea seems to explain an important reason why many women fail in their attempts to become slimmer and fitter, why so many feel deprived or—worse still—ill and debilitated on a diet they may have chosen. Just as there is no one perfect shape for everyone, there is no one diet for everyone.

Bel has been a consultant in personal development for six years with CMB, running her own consultancy in London. Her work has involved her in all aspects of personal presentation and appearance, including the analysis of individual body shapes, colouring and style.

She was aware of the need to help people to make the most of, and to come to terms with, their own individual body shape, and not aspire to unattainable ideals. It has particularly concerned her that most women she worked with were unhappy with some aspect of their bodies and most had been, or were on, a diet—the majority of them ultimately failing.

This book is the result of years of work and thought—and its message is, *we are not all the same*. Find *your* body shape and individual style, dietary and exercise needs—and your personal revolution has begun.

The Scientific Research

The scientific findings as to the significance of female body type are truly revolutionary. One of the early scientific papers which alerted other researchers to the correlation between body shape and metabolism was published in 1983 in the *Journal of Clinical Investigations* by researchers at the University of Gothenburg, Sweden. They divided 670 women into two basic body types; those who put weight on predominantly above the hips (this type of fat distribution follows the male pattern and so this type was called 'android') and those who put on weight predominantly on the lower hips, bottom and thighs (this is the traditional female pear shape, and so was called 'gynoid').

The researchers found that women with upper body adiposity had a predominance of large fat cells which reacted differently from the smaller fat cells characteristic of women with lower body adiposity. But most remarkably they found a significant increase in metabolic aberrations leading to diabetes and heart disease among the top-heavy android type compared with the bottom-heavy gynoid type.

'The principle is absolutely perfect. I felt really good. I wanted to lose 3–4.5 kg (7–10 lbs) and lost 4 kg (9 lbs) easily and quickly but what really amazed me is the loss in inches. Perhaps it's the combination of the foods. It was really important for me to realize how important exercise was. I now do a lot more on a regular basis. I have completely changed my exercise and eating habits.'

Nita
A TRIANGLE TYPE

In this Gothenburg paper's own words: 'The present study reports on extensive metabolic and morphologic investigations in 930 obese men and women. The data clearly showed that the men as a group were more susceptible than women to the metabolic aberrations induced by moderate obesity. *However, women with a typical male abdominal type of obesity, also had a metabolic risk profile resembling that of men.* When taken together, the results stressed the importance of the regional distribution of the adipose tissue to the metabolic aberrations that are seen in the obese state.'

The researchers believed that the most likely regulator of whether a

women is an 'android'- or a 'gynoid'-type is the sex-hormones. So it would seem that a gynoid-shaped woman's metabolism is more influenced by female hormones than the top-heavy android body shape, with male-type fat distribution. (And this might explain why, with the volunteer dieters, the Pear and Hourglass type women put on weight more readily from puberty onwards, although the Rectangle-type women caught up with them from their thirties onwards.)

A well-regarded paper published in 1982 from researchers at the Medical College of Wisconsin suggests that 'sites of fat distribution [in women] provide a diagnostic tool to predict abnormalities in glucose and lipid metabolism.' Most of these researchers use the ratio between waist measurement and hip measurement to determine whether a woman patient has a propensity of upper-body fat or lower-body fat (the closer the measurements are, the more 'apple-shaped' and therefore the more upper body fat: whereas a classic 'pear shape' will have a waist measurement significantly smaller than her hip measurement, an indication of lower-body fat).

'I feel really healthy and I've never eaten so much raw food and vegetables. Great. I am delighted with the whole thing.'

Jan
A PEAR TYPE

An interesting follow-up to the Gothenburg paper in 1984 suggests that women with increased upper-body fat should reduce their weight in order to reduce certain specific risks to their health. But it was recommended that further research was necessary to check the extent of this casual relationship: 'Our findings suggest that studies of reduction of body weight and concomitantly of the ratio of waist to hip circumference in subjects in whom this index is increased are urgently needed. The effect of such intervention should be studied with respect to risks for cardiovascular disease.'

An extensive paper published in 1988, 'A Weight Shape Index for Assessing Risk of Disease in 44,820 Women', extended the findings of the previous researchers. This study involved the researchers at the Medical College of Wisconsin again but this time with the collaboration of women on a sensible slimming programme with an American non-profit making slimming club. The women were divided into two age groups; 19,947 women in the 20–35 years group were investigated for correlation

between body fat distribution and menstrual abnormalities, and 24,873 women in the 40–59 years group were investigated for the prevalence of chronic diseases, diabetes, gall bladder and heart. The paper claimed: 'Upper-body fat predominance results in an increased risk of diabetes, hypertension, gallbladder disease and menstrual abnormalities.'

Dr Mary Loveday, Harley Street allergist and clinical ecologist, also recognises in her diagnostic work the significance of body shape. 'It is so necessary to realise that there is no ideal shape, and that we are born with a certain body type which is our lot. However, what we do (diet and exercise) can enhance that basic shape. I'm so sure that if we are unhappy with the quest for the "ideal" shape then that is the start of anorexia and bulimia.

'I too was intrigued by, and can verify that, the Triangle needs almost masculine exercise –whereas the Pears and Hourglasses hate it and need rather to do the gentle yoga.' Dr Loveday gave a warning that if a woman's basic body shape changes radically then medical opinion ought to be sought. For instance, a woman's thyroid can become over or under active, particularly at menopause, and can change a woman's natural pattern of weight distribution (when, for example, a natural Hourglass might lose her waist).

All women belong to one of four body shapes

Armed with these well-documented scientific facts, I was interested to see how they corresponded with my own findings about women and body shape. As a consultant on dressing and style, I had long recognized the two distinct female types described by the scientists. However, female body shape more accurately sub-divides again to make four classic types. Whether overweight or slim, young or old, any woman can be assigned to one of four body types: the 'Pear' and 'Hourglass' belong to the *gynoid* group and the 'Rectangle' and 'Triangle' belong to the *android* group. To further research the differences between these body types, I sent out 200 extensive questionnaires and the information from them has informed and reinforced the details of the four eating and exercise packages found in this book. One of the significant differences between body types,

which backs up the Swedish research of 1983 is that 100 per cent of the Pear-type women responding to the questionnaire said they put on weight, while less than 50 per cent of the Triangle type did (and they were seldom more than 3 kg [7 lbs] heavier than the weight they liked to be). Dr Loveday has also noticed this, pointing out that the gynoid shapes, the Pear and Hourglass, tend to put on more weight during pregnancy then the Rectangle- and Triangle-type women.

'Felt fitter after starting the diet. Once I started exercising at night I felt *even* fitter. The amount of food allowed per day is ideal.

Brilliant. Easy. I recommend it. . . '

Lindsay
AN HOURGLASS TYPE

Also with the aid of the questionnaire, I began to see that women with different body shapes appeared to have different attitudes towards dieting and exercise. One woman would say that dieting was not enough, she always had to exercise hard if she wanted a significant weight loss; another would insist that just cutting down on her food did all that was necessary and the most exercise she ever needed was a country walk or a bit of yoga, and that hard workouts in the gym were anathema.

Jenny Agutter, a famous 'gynoid' who swears by yoga, is one of these latter women: 'I've always hated aerobics and running, but there's something elegant about yoga.' And, in fact, it is the 'gynoid'-type women, the Pear- and Hourglass-shaped, who were more likely to be getting out of games at school, whereas the 'androids', the Rectangle- and Triangle-shaped women, remained the competitive, sporty types into adulthood. Think of all the leading women tennis players. Maria Bueno was the last gynoid champion and that was decades ago, before really hard-hitting 'masculine' play entered women's tennis.

Jane Fonda, who is on the opposite end of the body shape scale from Jenny Agutter, dedicated the second phase of her career to promoting really tough aerobic exercise for women. Ultimate physical fitness and stamina became a driving necessity for her in a way it never would for a gynoid-type woman. Not only do android-type women crave exercise, the evidence of the scientific papers outlined above would suggest that

they actually need to do aerobic exercise to help keep the arterial system healthy as android types are at greater risk of ill health when overweight than are gynoid-shaped women.

There is no one diet to suit everybody

We are bombarded with different diets, but all of them assume we are the same, that we have the same metabolisms and share the same dietary tastes and needs. Most work well for some people, but they do not work for everyone. Some faddy diets can be positively harmful.

In my work, women have expressed distinct differences in their success rate with various diets. The type of food which they ate and the time of eating have been significant factors in the success of a diet. In my experience, body type is also connected to the timing of our peaks of energy. It is better to eat your main meal when your metabolism is most active.

Dieticians have concluded that a diet will be more successful if a woman follows her natural eating and energy pattern. For instance, Rectangle-type women are more awake and active in the evening and therefore feel better and lose weight more efficiently if they have a very light breakfast, a light lunch and then their main meal at night.

That individuals have different dietary needs was made clear to me when I saw two clients, Jane and Christine, within a few days of each other. Both were on the same raw fruit and vegetable diet, but they had

'The diet was so easy to keep to, it actually re-educated my whole attitude to eating, so that I will stick to this system of eating permanently. I gained a lot of energy (as the 39-year-old mother of a two-and-three-quarter year old, a big bonus). I had no difficulty fitting the diet around my family—they adapted to the healthier system—I gave them extra helpings and they had potatoes added if requested. My little daughter and I developed a craving for fresh fruit. My husband loved the chick pea curry.

No calorie-counting was a boon— particularly when eating out. As a vegetarian it was easy to substitute a vegetarian product for the meat dishes.'

Diane
A RECTANGLE TYPE

responded very differently. Jane's skin was clearer, she said, than it had been for years: she felt light and full of energy and had lost 3 kg (7 lbs) in two weeks. Christine, on the other hand, was pale and lethargic. She said she felt dreadful and lacked energy and, worse still, did not seem to be losing weight significantly.

I knew that Jane and Christine were different body shapes (a Pear and Triangle respectively) and suggested Christine might try a diet with more protein. Her energy and well-being returned within two days and she started to lose weight.

There is no one ideal shape for everyone

It is sad but true that most women are dissatisfied with at least one part of their bodies and wish they could change it. We have images of 'perfect' female body shapes paraded before us from every medium: we grow up thinking there is one perfect type and most of us are convinced that if only we were not so greedy or lazy we could approximate to this ideal paraded in front of us by the fashion industry and Hollywood. The whole idea of an 'ideal' is made all the more impossible and ridiculous by the fact that it changes with the decades.

'This Pear diet and exercise programme is completely tuned into how I like to live. It makes absolute sense to me that we have different shapes and different metabolisms. I find this diet no hardship at all to follow and am delighted with how easily I have lost weight (6 kg [13 lbs] in six weeks) and how energetic and well I am looking and feeling. I think the whole body-type idea is fascinating and so obviously true. Thank you Bel.'

Jane
A PEAR TYPE

This is one of the most important messages of this book. I feel very strongly that by coming to terms with our shape, it is possible to make the most of it and *love* the body we have. That doesn't mean that we cannot be slimmer and trimmer and fitter generally, if we choose. But it does mean the end of unreasonable expectations and chronic dissatisfaction.

This realization has truly liberated me from the tyranny of the ideal body. The relief in knowing that no amount of exercise and dieting will produce a marked waist and board-flat tummy for me (a Rectangle type)

is tremendous. And it also helps me appreciate the good points about my body-type—slim legs, athletic build, strength and endurance. I know I cannot be the typical model-girl shape (Triangle) or a curvy siren shape like Marilyn Monroe or Joan Collins (Hourglass) but I can make the most of what I am. AND SO CAN YOU.

163 kg (358 lbs) in 6 weeks!

The scientific facts and anecdotal evidence helped me formulate an extensive, in-depth questionnaire on dietary and exercise needs which I sent out to 200 women. The results from this gave me the basis for the four body-type diet and exercise programmes. To refine these further, I asked for volunteer dieters to follow the programme designed for their individual body-type for six weeks (some continued much longer). Their experiences and comments helped make the four body-type programmes in this book tailor-made for you.

The progress of these dieters was fantastic. Thirty women divided into the four basic types lost 163 kg (358 lbs) in six weeks! That's an average of nearly 5.5 kg (12 lbs) per person which delighted them and me. Some only had a few kilos to lose (as you can see in the weight and measurement chart with each body-type package), but there were others who had a long way to go. It was they who particularly touched me by their progress: women who had never managed to lose so much before on *any* diet; women who had lost more than 12.5 kg (2 stone) in those six weeks, and those who were lighter than they had been for 20 years.

All these women's lives and spirits were enhanced by their sense of achievement, their greater energy and their pleasure in their looks. And all of them, now months later, have continued to lose weight or maintain their new weight, all saying they have learned a better way of eating *for them* which will be a healthy plan for life.

We had great fun during the six-week experiment. Only two women dropped out, and both for good personal reasons. Everyone else showed such enthusiasm and success that all the hard work of thinking out and planning these programmes was rewarded many times over. Some personal anecdotes of the volunteer dieters are included in each diet and exercise package. It has been a marvellous experience and I am very

grateful indeed to all those women whose experiences, suggestions and—best of all—successes have helped me make this book.

Everything that I've learnt about body shape and its significance in all aspects of life, particularly on diet and exercise, is here in this book. My own experience, the experiences of my family, friends and clients, and the scientific papers have all contributed. Now that you've done the questionnaire and discovered your own body type you have the key to your own transformation. Today is the first day of the rest of your life—join us and start now.

•When I read your introduction to the Hourglass body type I really felt that you were speaking to me personally, almost that you could see into my mind. It was so me.

I didn't feel like I was on a diet. The cottage cheese and fruit for lunch suited me greatly and I've gladly had it every day for eight weeks. Also the chick pea curry was delicious.

I've bought a new leotard to replace my usual baggy top.•

Denise
AN HOURGLASS TYPE

References

Kissebah, Ahmed H. et al., 1982: Relation of Body Fat Distribution to Metabolic Complications of Obesity. *Journal of Clinical Endocrinology and Metabolism*. Vol. 54, No.2, pp. 254–259.

Krotkiewski, Marcin et al., 1983: Impact of Obesity on Metabolism in Men & Women: Importance of Regional Adipose Tissue Distribution. *Journal of Clinical Investigations*. Vol. 72, September 1983, pp. 1150–1162.

Lapidus, Leif et al., 1984: Distribution of Adipose Tissue and Risk of Cardiovascular Disease and Death: a 12 year follow up of participants in the population study of women in Gothenburg, Sweden. *British Medical Journal*. Vol. 289, 10th November 1984, pp. 1257–1261.

Alfred A. Rimm, Arthur J. Hartz and Mary E. Fischer, 1988: A Weight Shape Index for Assessing Risk of Disease in 44,820 Women. *Journal of Clinical Epidemiology*. Vol. 41, No. 5, pp. 459–465, 1988.

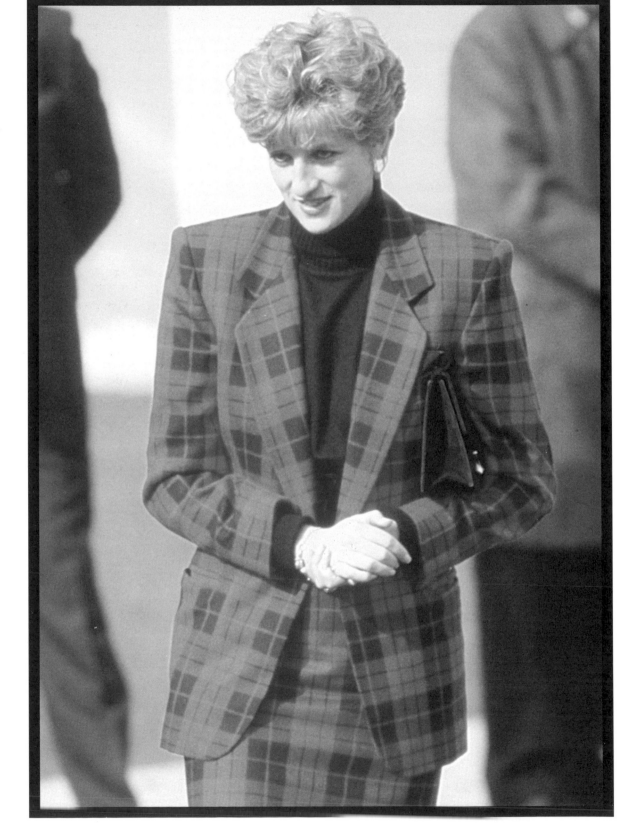

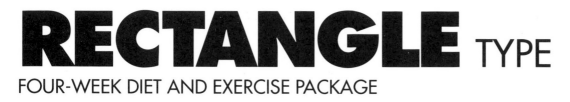

RECTANGLE TYPE
FOUR-WEEK DIET AND EXERCISE PACKAGE

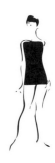

THIS IS a four-week package of diet menus and exercise programmes tailor-made for your body-type and metabolism. A team of volunteer dieters tested this diet and exercise programme for six weeks, some for three months and more. Their experiences and comments went into improving it for you. With each week, my volunteer dieters and I found it was very encouraging to have a treat, or 'positive action' as it came to be known, to lift our spirits and keep us going through the next week. As you read through the package you will see what I mean.

Individual characteristics

The Rectangle type has a robust constitution. She has an athletic body with a strength and solidity about it which is mirrored in the constancy of her energy flow. Because of her big appetite and balanced body shape, the Rectangle type can get very overweight indeed in her middle and later years. This is when our sporty youth has given way to more sedentary middle-age, but our appetites remain.

The Rectangle type tends to be a late-in-the-day type who, if she isn't being forced to get up really early by children or work demands, would naturally be a late starter who then works, or parties, into the night. This type positively *needs* regular, energetic exercise and can get depressed if she isn't doing any. She is at her best when doing regular aerobic exercise, ie exercise which raises the heart rate, like aerobics, speed swimming, jogging, bicycling.

This type finds it hard to stop eating once she starts and so needs a diet with some restraining boundaries. (I know because I am one.) There is plenty of anecdotal evidence that greater health and weight loss can be achieved by not mixing food in one meal which is a concentrated carbohydrate with food that is concentrated protein, eg meat with vegetable and salad is fine but meat with bread or potatoes is wrong mixing.

Princess Diana is a classic Rectangle. Sporty as a girl, prone to put on weight on her tummy and upper torso when not exercising, this type is a marvellous clothes-horse when slim like Princess Diana. Her fashion sense has evolved over the years and now she rarely gets her style wrong. This suit is excellent in that it follows the line of her body, square shoulders, straight jacket, little waist-shaping and a narrow, tapering skirt. The bold check fabric too suits her angular shape but ideally the lapels and jacket hem should be straight.

The Rectangle type is a shape Princess Diana shares with her mother-in-law and grandmother-in-law—although on a different scale. Exercise is necessary for this type, and with the scientific findings (see Science section, page 16) it is important not just for reasons of looking good but for health and general well-being.

RECTANGLE

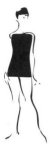

RECTANGLE-TYPE WEIGHT AND MEASUREMENTS BEFORE DIETING, AND SIX WEEKS LATER

| | WEIGHT (kg/st & lbs) | | MEASUREMENTS (cms/ins) | | | | | |
| | | | BEFORE | | | AFTER | | |
NAME	BEFORE	AFTER	BUST	WAIST	HIPS	BUST	WAIST	HIPS
Ruth	107/17 0	97.5/15 7	127.5/51	117.5/47	135/54	117.5/47	109/43½	130/52
Barbara	72.5/11 7	68.5/10 12	102.5/41	87.5/35	105/42	99/39½	80/32	100/40
Karen	66.5/10 8	60.5/9 8	97.5/39	82.5/33	95/38	94/37½	75/30	94/37½
Linda	74/11 10	71/11 4	102.5/41	86/34½	106/42½	100/40	80/32	100/40
Chris	98/15 8	85/13 7	114/45½	110/44	127.5/51	105/42	100/40	117.5/47
Elyse	82/13 0	76.5/12 2	111/44½	90/36	114/45½	104/41½	85/34	105/42
Marthe	60/9 7	57.5/9 2	85/34	67.5/27	84/33½	85/34	65.5/26¼	82.5/33
Diane	71.5/11 5	66/10 7	97.5/39	90/36	104/41½	97.5/39	80/32	99/39½

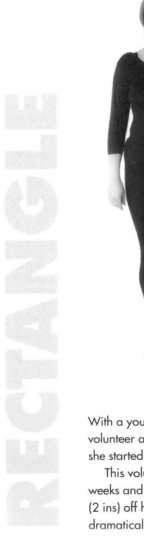

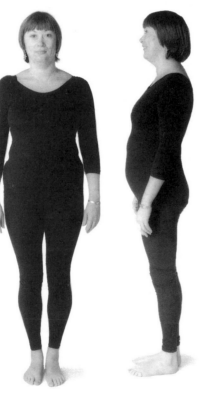

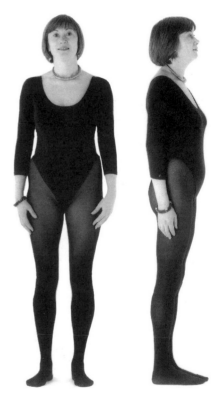

BEFORE

AFTER

With a young daughter and a teaching job, our volunteer above had little time for exercise but when she started the Rectangle-type diet, she made time.

This volunteer lost a total of 5.5 kg (12 lbs) in six weeks and lost 10 cms (4 ins) off her waist and 5 cms (2 ins) off her hips. Her weight loss can be seen most dramatically in profile, with her spare tyre, tummy and

upper back markedly flatter. Unlike the Hourglass and Pear types, Rectangles get deeper when they put on weight, and nothing demonstrates this better than her 'before' photo. It is typical also for a Rectangle to noticeably put on weight—and lose it—in the face and neck area, and it is good to see this volunteer's face so much lighter.

RECTANGLE

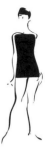

RECTANGLE-TYPE DIETERS' WEIGHT LOSS OVER SIX WEEKS (kg/lbs)

NAME	WEEK:	1	2	3	4	5	6	TOTAL WEIGHT LOSS
Ruth		4/9	1.4/3	0.9/2	0.9/2	0.9/2	1.4/3	−9.5/21
Barbara		0.9/2	1.4/3	0.5/1	0/0	0.5/1	0.9/2	−4/9
Karen		3.1/7	1.4/3	0.5/1	1.4/3	0.9/2	+0.9/2	−6.3/14
Linda		1.4/3	0/0	+0.5/1	0.5/1	1.4/3	0/0	−2.7/6
Chris		6.3/14	0.9/2	2.7/6	1.6/3½	1.6/3½	0/0	−13/29
Elyse		1.4/3	1.4/3	0.5/1	0.9/2	0.5/1	0.9/2	−5.5/12
Marthe		0.9/2	2.2/5	0/0	+0.5/1	0.5/1	+0.9/2	−2.2/5
Diane		0.9/2	1.8/4	0.5/1	1.8/4	0.5/1	0/0	−5.5/12

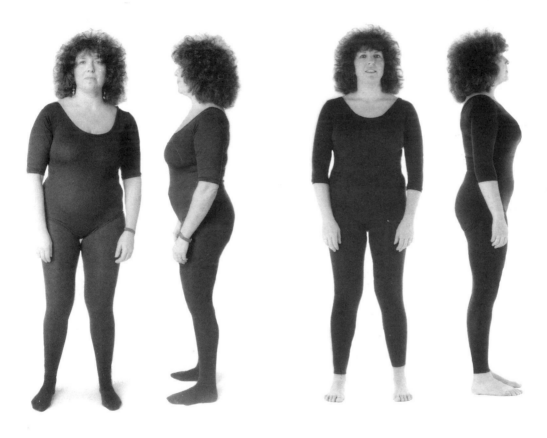

BEFORE

AFTER

Our volunteer above also lost 5.5 kg (12 lbs) in six weeks, together with 7.5 cms (3 ins) off her bust, 5 cms (2 ins) off her waist and 7.5 cms (3 ins) off her hips. Again her face and upper chest area look much

slimmer. Because the Rectangle type so readily puts on weight on her face, it is marvellous to see that this volunteer's weight loss is reflected in her face, making her look years younger.

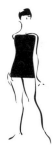

WEEK ONE
Positive action: enhance your style

AS YOU'VE already seen, we don't all share the same body shape and an outfit that looks fantastic on one person can look dreadful on somebody else. And this is not just a matter of slenderness. Wearing clothes which suit your body shape, drawing attention to your good points and hiding your not so good, can give you the appearance of having *lost 3 kg (7 lbs)* before you even begin your diet.

With a Rectangle-type body, your hips and shoulders are similar in width and you do not have a marked waist. Princess Diana, Vanessa Redgrave, Maureen Lipman and Glenn Close are slim versions of this type; Victoria Wood, Cilla Black and Jennifer Saunders the more generous examples. Unlike the Pear and Hourglass, your hips are not curvy but straight and when you put on weight you become 'deeper' rather than wider, more a cube than a rectangle. Your legs remain slimmer than the rest of you, however heavy you get.

The basic principle of style is that you wear clothes which have the same or similar line to your body line. So jackets and tops look better if they are straight cut, without a marked waist and no curvy details in seams and lapels. Square shoulders suit you better than curved and you need clothes which look as if they've been well-tailored in a good fabric. Keep to the crisp strong fabrics like gaberdine, worsted wools, heavy silks. Crumpled linens and thin silks, which suit the Pear and Hourglass, can just look messy and unbecoming on you.

Skirts and trousers are much more flattering to this shape if they continue this geometrical look, straight and tapering to the hem. There should be no pleating or gathering into the waistband. Keep the profile straight and lean.

Scooped necklines are not flattering to this shape so keep to shirt style, boat, square or V-necks. Flimsy fabrics like organza, chiffon, soft silks and lace are too soft and can look frumpy or cheap on you. Unless you have straight shoulders, square shoulder pads in everything from jackets to T-shirts add elegance and sharpness to your style. Keep all your clothes and accessory detail geometrical rather than curvy—necklines, lapels and jacket edges, belt buckles and handbags.

Good shoes and accessories and an important piece of geometric jewellery will help give your business dressing a chic and crisp look.

If you are very overweight

If this is the case, these general style pointers need a bit of modification. There is a tendency for overweight women to try to camouflage everything and some end up wearing a tent in despair. But all shapes, even carrying a lot of extra weight, still have their distinctive good points and clothes should show these to advantage.

Most of the Rectangle type's extra weight is in the upper body area, on tummy, bust and shoulders. Your lower hips and legs remain relatively slim and so it is best if you keep to straight skirts and trousers. If you feel you need a more roomy skirt make sure it retains its straight lines with crisp pleats and a non-crease fabric. Flares and gathers will only make you look heavier.

Your jackets too should keep their straight lines, no waists, peplums, rounded hems or lapels, and hang onto your shoulder pads to keep your shoulder line crisp. You may feel, however, that your jackets have a more flattering line, especially if you have a big bust, if they are in softer materials than suggested in the general guidelines. Rather than gaberdine, for instance, wear soft wools and cottons, or a good quality silk. But, as with the general advice for your shape, keep away from linens and other fabrics which crease badly, as these will only make you look untidy.

It may also be more flattering to your shape if you wear longer length jackets—if you have the height. A straight dress with a straight three-quarter length jacket can be remarkably slimming. However overweight you are, remember that the best profile for you is broad at the top and narrower at the bottom. Anything with a waist or a full skirt is going to look frumpy on you. Your lower legs are likely to remain slim and should be emphasized. Even if you think you're too big for this narrow profile dressing do just try a straight, knee-length or just below

knee-length skirt, or narrow-legged trousers, with a loose tunic top. You will be amazed to find how flattering this look can be to all variations within this Rectangle body type.

A more youthful and informal variation of this look is an oversize sweater in a good colour or pattern, or a large shirt in a crisp, strong material, worn over good quality (non-baggy) leggings. Even in casual dress like this, square shoulder pads rather than round help me look slimmer and more angular.

RECTANGLE

29

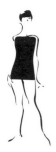

WEEK ONE

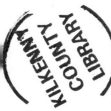
RECTANGLE

Jewellery

Jewellery for the Rectangle type should, like her clothes, follow the line of her body. Keep it geometrical rather than curvy. Chain link bracelets and necklaces are better as flat, geometric links—like brick-link —rather than curvy curb-link.

Because you tend to put weight on your face and neck, if you like wearing necklaces keep away from the choker-length, which can make you look thick in the neck, and go for a more flattering longer length to wear over blouses or tops. Bold chain necklaces are good, but if you want beads, go for those with more geometrical detail. This visual effect of angularity can result from the way the beads are linked or, for instance, if they are threaded with strips of straight bone or metal, or have similar straight insets between them. The beads themselves can be less than perfectly round, some even square or rectangular.

Brooches for the Rectangle type are best if they have a predominance of straight lines. One of my favourite brooches is a painted 7.5cm (3in) square, with one of its corners cut off. It is simple, but

because it suits me so perfectly in line and scale (I am large boned and need big jewellery) it looks really classy.

Do remember, *scale* is as important in jewellery as it is in clothes. It has to be the right size for you. If you are large boned (as a rough guide if your wrist measures 16.5cms [6½ins] or more) then your jewellery pieces ought to be large and important. If you are medium (14 to 16.5cms [5½ to 6½ins]) to small boned (less than 14cms [5½ins]) then make sure your jewellery does not overwhelm you.

Watches look better on you if they have oblong or square faces with straight straps or bracelets. Some of the more elegant men's watches can be perfect in style and scale—unless you are very petite and small boned when you're better off with something more delicate but still geometric.

So, as your first positive action, make yourself feel better and look slimmer in the right clothes and accessories for your shape. Then with this boost to your image start on the first week of your tailor-made diet and exercise plan and begin to lose pounds of *real* weight.

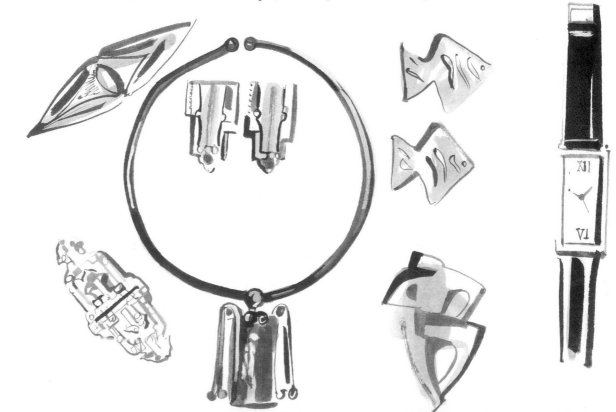

30

Starting your diet

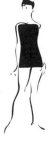

This is a low-fat diet. With a reduced fat, reduced sugar and increased fibre intake, this diet takes into account the latest findings on healthy nutrition. It also incorporates the basic principles of not mixing carbohydrates and proteins in one meal (vegetables, other than potatoes, are neutral and can be eaten in unlimited quantity with either type of meal). At least four hours should be allowed to elapse between each meal to allow complete digestion to take place.

The menus which follow are for those of you who like a structured diet. For the rest, they are suggestions for meals based on the basic principles of your body-type diet of lean protein (fish, unfatty meat, eggs), unrefined carbohydrates (like baked potato, wholemeal bread, brown rice), with almost limitless salad and vegetables, and generous amounts of fruit. The Rectangle type's metabolism responds better to a diet that provides at least one substantial meal a day, ideally in the evening, otherwise you begin to feel deprived and rebellious. With your regular aerobic exercise routine you will increase your metabolic rate and therefore are allowed a few more calories in your diet than the more sedentary body types.

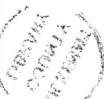

You can switch meals around from day to day— or repeat easy or favourite ones—as long as you have lunches at lunchtime and suppers in the evening. Useful, though not ideal, if you are too busy, or disinclined to cook, are the ready-made, low-calorie frozen meals. You may substitute these for your main meal but add a salad or vegetables. This diet should not only help the Rectangle type to lose weight but to be healthier, look better and feel great.

This diet does not allow for alcohol. There are two main reasons for this: alcohol represents empty calories and I would rather you got food value for your extra calories in the shape of an extra piece of fruit, or another helping of salad or vegetables—or even a slightly larger helping of protein: fish or eggs or chicken. But most importantly, alcohol undermines our self-control—and can be addictive. Once we've had one drink it's much easier to have another, and then our resolve goes and we're eating anything that comes our way.

It's much easier and generally more efficient if you can cut out alcohol for the duration of your diet. Many women find that they can lose weight just by

---

DAILY ALLOWANCE

300 ml (½ pt) skimmed milk
15 g (½ oz) low-fat spread

Beverages: try to keep your intake of tea/coffee to two cups a day, but drink plenty of water and have as many cups of herb tea as you like

Unlimited vegetables (preferably raw, otherwise boiled/steamed):

asparagus	aubergine	bean sprouts	beetroot
broccoli	brussel sprouts	cabbage	carrots
cauliflower	celery	chard	chicory
courgettes	cucumbers	French beans	endive
escarole	green/red pepper	kale	lettuce
mange-tout peas	mushrooms	okra	onions
parsley	radishes	runner beans	spinach
spring greens	tomatoes	turnips	watercress

Permitted fruits where indicated (no snacking!):

apple	apricot	handful blackberries	grapefruit
kiwi	nectarine	orange	peach
pear	plum	tangerine	watermelon, 1 slice

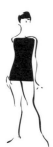

WEEK ONE

doing this, so unaware were they of how many extra calories they were consuming every day in liquid form.

However, I am aware that for some women this is an impossibility and if it is the difference between going on the diet or not, obviously I would rather you follow the dieting guidelines and limit your alcohol to one drink a day, preferably with your meal.

For vegetarians there are recipes for main meal substitutions in the recipe supplement on pages 72–9.

DAY ONE
Breakfast
40 g (1½ oz) unsweetened muesli, bran flakes, puffed wheat or any other unsweetened breakfast cereal, (with skimmed milk from daily allowance), cup tea or coffee.
Lunch
Quick pea soup (see recipe, on page 76) or 300 ml (½ pt) non-creamy packet soup (lentil/vegetable), one piece wholemeal bread, banana, cup of tea.
Supper
225 g (8 oz) white fish, grilled or steamed, green salad (as much as you like), low-cal dressing, either commercial brand or home-made (see recipe, on page 72), two-fruit salad, 1 tbsp low-fat natural yogurt.

DAY TWO
Breakfast
Two pieces wholemeal toast, low-fat spread from daily allowance, cup of tea or coffee.
Lunch
One hard-boiled egg, 25 g (1 oz) feta cheese chopped into large mixed salad (from permitted list), creamy low-cal dressing (see recipe, page 72), cup of tea.
Supper
Tandoori chicken (see recipe, page 76), big salad or selection of vegetables (from permitted list), baked apple cooked with two chopped dried apricots as stuffing, 1 tbsp frozen yogurt

DAY THREE
Breakfast
Either as Day 1 or Day 2.
Lunch
Bean and lentil salad (see recipe, page 75), 150 g (5 oz) low-fat fruit yogurt, cup of tea.
Supper
175 g (6 oz) fresh (grilled) or tinned tuna (in brine not oil), steamed vegetables (from permitted list), fresh fruit salad (from permitted list).

DAY FOUR
Breakfast
Either as Day 1 or Day 2.

‘I can't believe it. I don't feel ravenously hungry, I'm not grumpy and tired, I'm not planning some binge when the trial comes to an end *and* my digestive system, which has always been quirky, is working more calmly and efficiently than ever before. It's almost too much to hope that I'm losing weight as well, but I am. Oh, and in my new leggings and tunic top I look a stone lighter already.’

Barbara

RECTANGLE

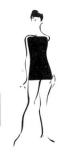

Lunch
Mushroom omelette (see recipe, page 76), mixed salad, low-cal dressing (see recipe, page 72) or steamed vegetables, mango or any two fruits from permitted list.

Supper
Spaghetti with broccoli (see recipe, page 74), baked pepper salad (see recipe, page 77), one slice of wholemeal bread, banana split (1 tbsp iced vanilla yogurt instead of ice cream).

DAY FIVE
Breakfast
Either as Day 1 or Day 2.

Lunch
150 g (5 oz) cottage cheese mixed with chopped olives, radishes, spring onions, green salad, apple, cup of tea.

Supper
175 g (6 oz) rump steak grilled, steamed green vegetables (from permitted list), orange.

DAY SIX
Breakfast
Either as Day 1 or Day 2.

Lunch
Tabbouleh (see recipe, page 77) in wholemeal pitta bread, small bunch of grapes, cup of tea.

Supper
Salade Niçoise (see recipe, page 76), one slice of wholemeal bread, glass unsweetened fruit juice.

DAY SEVEN
Breakfast
Either as Day 1 or Day 2.

Lunch
Baked potato, 110 g (4 oz) baked beans, large green salad, low-cal dressing (see recipe, page 72), cup of tea.

Supper
225 g (8 oz) white fish baked, steamed or grilled, tomato and onion salad, on bed of lettuce, low-cal dressing (see recipe, page 72), 50 g (2 oz) prunes, stewed, 1 tbsp low-fat natural yogurt.

'The effect on body shape has been amazing—in the first six weeks I lost 5.5 kg (12 lbs) and still lose 1 kg (2 lbs) weekly on average—I am going on until I reach 63 kg (10 stone). Just 2.7 kg (6 lbs) to go.

The most staggering improvement has been in the severe fluid retention problem I suffered for up to two weeks out of four during my menstrual cycle. I would bloat up by 3 kg (7 lbs) and the extra fluid caused so much pressure on my joints that my GP actually tested me for arthritis. After the first week of the diet I felt full of energy. By the end of week two I braced myself for the big bloat but a miracle had happened. My weight remained stable. I put on only 0.5 kg (1 lb) during the whole of my period this month.'

Diane

RECTANGLE

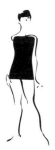

WEEK ONE
Your exercise programme

The Rectangle type is naturally athletic, with a powerful body which positively needs to be exercised vigorously. Aerobic sports like jogging, speed swimming, competitive squash and tennis, are best suited to this type's physique and temperament. If you are seriously overweight, or haven't exercised for ages, get medical advice first and start off slowly, walking briskly and swimming, building up over two weeks to the more vigorous sports.

I cannot stress enough how important it is for this type to combine any diet with an exercise regime. Exercise is an essential part of an efficient weight-loss programme for the Rectangle and she should aim to stick to it if she can. She should do some sort of aerobic activity at least three times a week, for at least half an hour each time. This not only burns calories (half an hour of speed swimming or squash will use up 300 calories) but it raises the metabolic rate for a few hours after as well.

❝I've always known that I need to exercise in order to feel good and keep slim—just dieting has never really worked for me. So on your programme I have taken up aerobics, do your excellent exercises (which are working away at my solid waist) and have changed my eating habits. I am feeling and looking like a New Woman (it's done wonders for my self esteem).❞

Isabel

There is also a 'feel good' factor to exercising which cannot be over-emphasized. If you're doing the exercise that suits your body type and disposition it undoubtedly lifts the spirits, makes you generally more positive about yourself, more in tune with your body—and less likely to neglect and abuse it.

When I realized how important exercise was to my type's health, slimness and well-being my heart sank. I didn't want to have to be so organized and self-disciplined. I had got into the bad habit of doing hardly any exercise and what I did I would do in a mad rush, like swimming flat out until I was exhausted, and then not do anything for the next few weeks. I felt sluggish and depressed.

But deep down I knew that a regular exercise regime was what I really needed. It was the only way I could efficiently lose weight. It also made me feel *so much better* and more energetic in everything else I did. Now, doing half an hour of uninterrupted power swimming three times a week makes the most dramatic difference to my mood, my efficiency—and my shape. The tummy, which most Rectangles have a battle with, is distinctly toned up—although I am resigned to the fact that it will never be as flat as that of my naturally Pear-type friend.

So I'm afraid there's no avoiding the fact that this type needs and thrives on hard exercise, from figure, mood and health points of view. Join that tennis club, that aerobics class, that marathon training. Or just make sure you run to work three times a week. Anything to get your heart working and the metabolism burning. The great consolation is to think of how good you're going to feel—and also, don't forget that 300 calories are burnt for every really energetic half-hour's exercise.

As flexibility in the waist area can be a problem for us Rectangle shapes I have included two floor exercises to be done every day which will tackle this immobility, and strengthen and tone the tummy muscles. This type tends to find floor exercises rather too inactive and boring so I am not giving you as many to do as the curvy shapes, but it is in the expectation that you will be taking up some active aerobic exercise instead.

Waist mobility swing

1 Sit on the floor, right foot bent back behind you, and left foot tucked under your right thigh. Keep your back straight.

2 Push your left hip into the floor as you slowly raise your arms above your head, stretching up as far as you can, *lifting from the waist.*

3 Bend your body to the right as you swing your arms down in the same direction. Make sure your movement swings to the side rather than towards the front, to get maximum stretch on those side muscles.

4 Swing your arms back to above your head and then lower them to your sides. *Repeat the movement five times.*

5 Change position to the other side; left foot back behind you, right foot tucked under your left thigh. Then repeat the movements, keeping your back straight and swing to the side, not towards the front of your body. REPEAT EXERCISE FIVE TIMES.

Stomach and waist trimmer

This is an exercise which has a vigorous effect on the muscles of the stomach. You must do it carefully and accurately so that it does not strain your back at all. The moment your back hurts you should stop, a sign that you are not using your stomach muscles properly. Follow the instructions carefully.

1 Lie flat on your back on a carpet or folded blanket, with your knees bent and your feet tucked under a bed or sofa, and hands by your side.

2 Tighten your buttock muscles and round your shoulders and stretch your arms forwards. Making sure your back is *pressed* into the floor, slowly pull yourself up until your body is quarter-sitting, curled forwards towards your knees and looking a little like a cradle. *Keep the small of your back on the floor all the time.*

3 Thinking of your tummy muscles as strong bands of elastic, reach forward and then move slightly back. *Repeat the whole gentle movement to and fro three times.*

4 Uncurl your spine and slowly lower your upper back and shoulders to the floor. Press the small of your back into the carpet. REPEAT EXERCISE THREE TIMES.

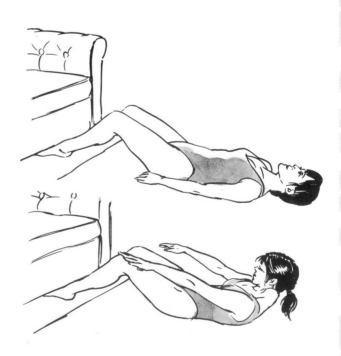

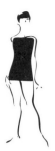

WEEK TWO
Positive action: instant healthy glow

GO AND buy yourself a blusher. Nothing lifts the contours of a face and the colour of a complexion more immediately and naturally than blusher. Buy a powder in a neutral rosy tone and apply it as shown in the illustration below.

1 Brush blush along the cheekbone, starting on a level with the outer edge of your iris and feathering it upwards and outwards as far as the hairline at the top of your ear.

2 You might like also to add the slightest touch of colour to your temples and chin.

3 Blend the edges with a soft powder brush. Never have definite lines in any make-up you apply.

The sporty Rectangle type of woman quite often will say to me that she doesn't use make-up. It usually means she is not confident about using it and doesn't like a made-up look. My answer is that from our mid-twenties onwards our colouring tends to fade and the definition of our features softens with age. I never advocate a stagey effect, but do point out that if you are in business, well-applied and sub-tle make-up gives your features greater definition and adds more authority to your whole image.

If you still feel reluctant or lacking in competence, try using just your new blusher and a soft neutral lipstick and see if you like the effect. This should make your complexion brighter, your eyes more intense in colour and your face more contoured.

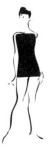

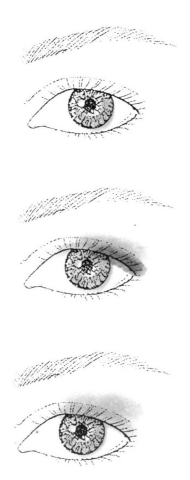

1 Highlighter: using an eye-shadow sponge, apply a light, neutral colour on the whole area of your upper eye from eyelid to brow.

2 Lid: apply a light to medium colour just on the lid (a taupe or soft olive suit most people), blending with a small brush.

3 Orbital bone: apply a darker colour along the upper eye-socket crease, blending it onto the lid at the outer corner of the eye. Blend all the colours with a soft brush. The end result must look like a wash of colour over your lid, getting darker towards the socket and the outside edge. No stripes or hard edges please.

4 Mascara: finish the look off with a couple of coats of brown mascara on the upper lashes, and one coat on the lower.

Subtly applied eye make-up needs a bit more technique and practice. But it is eye make-up which most fair-skinned, light-eyelashed women particularly feel they need. In my classes, even the most tentative women manage a professional job after experimenting for half an hour. Without being able to advise you personally, taking into account your individual colouring and shape of eye, I can only give the steps which are outlined and illustrated above as a general pointer.

Rectangle types tend to put on weight on their faces and shoulders so by now you may be noticing that your first week's dieting has already begun to reveal more marked cheekbones and a cleaner jaw-line—and a longer, slimmer neck. There is something very satisfying about rediscovering your younger, more clearly defined face. Certainly, on this diet your skin will improve—although you may find that during the first week it's a bit spotty as you clear some of the toxins out of your system.

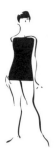

WEEK TWO
Your diet

DAY EIGHT

Breakfast
40 g (1½ oz) unsweetened muesli, bran flakes, puffed wheat or any other unsweetened breakfast cereal, (with skimmed milk from daily allowance), cup of tea or coffee.

Lunch
100 g (4 oz) peeled prawns, large mixed salad, creamy low-cal dressing (see recipe, page 72), orange, cup of tea.

Supper
Ratatouille (see recipe, page 74) with 50 g (2 oz) rice (dry weight, preferably brown) boiled, ginger banana (see recipe, page 79).

DAY NINE

Breakfast
Two pieces of wholemeal toast, low-fat spread from daily allowance, cup tea or coffee.

Lunch
100 g (4 oz) cottage cheese, apple and orange chopped in, cup of tea.

Supper
175 g (6 oz) chicken breast, rubbed with 1 tsp olive oil and herbs, grilled, selection of vegetables (from permitted list), baked apple cooked with two dried apricots as stuffing, 1 tbsp low-fat natural yogurt.

DAY TEN

Breakfast
Either as Day 8 or Day 9.

Lunch
300 ml (½ pt) any non-creamy packet soup or homemade vegetable soup (see recipe, page 75), one piece of wholemeal bread/toast, banana, cup of tea.

⁶It is wonderful having the main large meal of the day in the evening as a reward. This means you can go out to dinner and be able to really eat something instead of just pretending all you really wanted was the lettuce garnish. It really suits the way I live and work. Having to eat my main meal in the middle of the day would have been impossible. It meant I didn't have to start adapting the diet from day one which is always fatal.

The licence to eat loads of the permitted vegetables was great. You could really fill your plate. On other diets I have tried they advise you to use a smaller plate, etc, which never helped. On this diet you can have a heaped plate of salad which helps psychologically.

I never felt hungry on the diet and I have lost more weight than I ever thought possible.⁹

Ruth

RECTANGLE

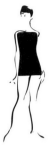

Supper

200 g (7 oz) smoked haddock, steamed or poached in skimmed milk (from daily allowance) and water, two or more vegetables (from permitted list), one piece of fruit cut into 150 g (5 oz) low-fat natural yogurt.

DAY ELEVEN

Breakfast

Either as Day 8 or Day 9.

Lunch

Spanish omelette (see recipe, page 76), green salad, low-cal dressing (see recipe, page 72), one piece of fruit (from permitted list).

Supper

Chick pea curry (see recipe, page 74), 25 g (1 oz) rice (dry weight, preferably brown) boiled, banana split with 1 tbsp frozen natural yogurt instead of ice cream.

DAY TWELVE

Breakfast

Either as Day 8 or Day 9.

Lunch

100 g (4 oz) cottage cheese, baked pepper and anchovy (see recipe, page 77), one piece of fruit, cup of tea.

Supper

Mixed grill of two back rashers bacon (all fat trimmed off), one lamb's kidney, two small low-fat sausages, tomatoes, mushrooms (all grilled, not fried), green side salad, low-cal dressing (see recipe, page 72), 150 g (5 oz) low-fat natural yogurt, chopped apple, few raisins.

DAY THIRTEEN

Breakfast

Either as Day 8 or Day 9.

Lunch

Baked potato, 1 tbsp hummus, mixed salad, low-cal dressing (see recipe, page 72), 150 g (5 oz) low-fat fruit yogurt, cup of tea.

Supper

Kyoto trout salad (see recipe, page 75), stewed prunes and apricots (two of each), 1 tbsp frozen natural yogurt.

DAY FOURTEEN

Breakfast

Either as Day 8 or Day 9.

Lunch

Three fruits (from permitted list) made into fruit salad with 150 g (5 oz) low-fat natural yogurt or 75 g (3 oz) fromage frais (8% fat), cup of tea.

Supper

Quarter of chicken, grilled or dry roasted, large mixed salad, low-cal dressing (see recipe, page 72), one piece of fruit.

Your exercise programme

Increase the repetitions of the floor exercises as outlined in the box below.

I hope that you have been able to organize your life around some regular exercise and are beginning to feel the benefits. Certainly the mental advantage cannot be overlooked. A sense of well-being and good spirits, and pleasure in your active and increasingly fit body all help to reinforce the positive effects of this programme. Keeping your spirits up also helps to maintain the resolve to continue with the programme and eventually to integrate exercise and sensible eating into your life.

EXERCISE PROGRAMME: WEEK TWO	
Waist Mobility Swing	7
Stomach and Waist Trimmer	4

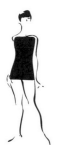

WEEK THREE
Positive action: good foundations

YOU ARE due for a reward for having got this far and lost those first pounds—some of you may be as much as 3 kg (7 lbs) lighter by this point, others more like 1.8–2.3 kg (4–5 lbs). Whatever weight you have lost, you will notice a flattening of the bulges. You may well feel like treating yourself to an indulgence that does not involve food. I suggest the luxury of a new piece of underwear which will make you feel pampered and proud of your body.

Women with straight hips are more flattered by sporty underwear and Rectangle types are practical women who like to be comfortable. Cotton, no frills, high-cut legs are just right for you. Those high-cut sporty underpants are comfortable and sexy on your straight-limbed body. Any lace insets should be stiffish rather than flimsy. This is one body shape which an all-in-one doesn't generally flatter.

This body type often has big, rather low breasts. A good quality underwired bra will be comfortable and give you good support. If you feel like a bit of lace, keep it to a half cup. At night or for lounging around, your shape looks very good in mansize pyjamas—no frilly baby dolls for you. So go ahead and spoil yourself —make it silk!

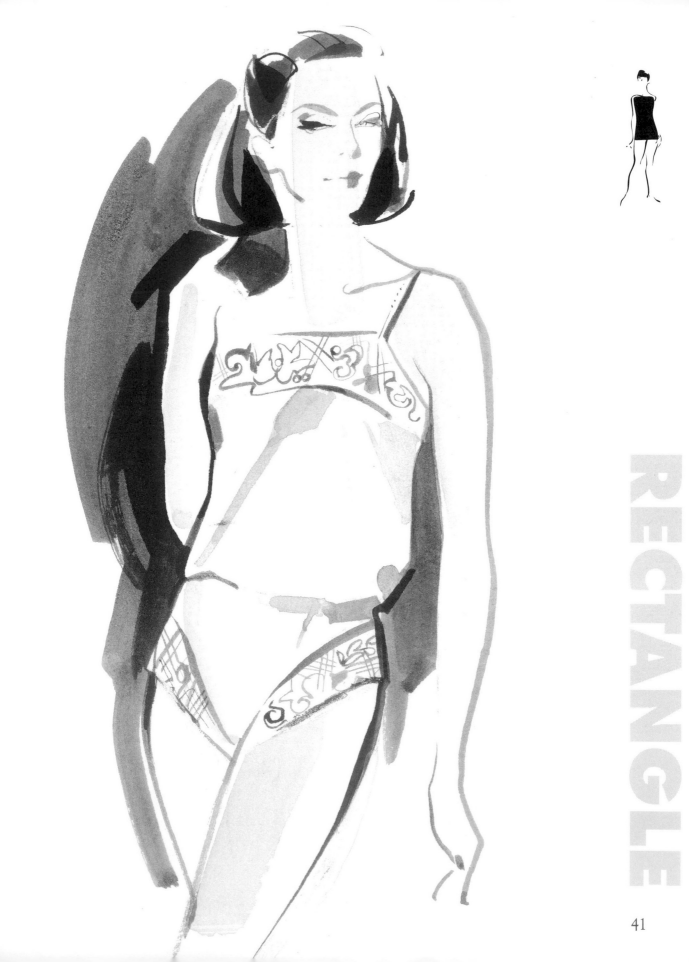

RECTANGLE

41

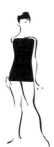

WEEK THREE
Your diet

This week can be a danger week. I found with my volunteer dieters that this could be the one when they lost heart. Weight loss having been really good in the first two weeks now tends to slow down. Boredom or resentment at not being able to eat your favourite foods may ambush all your good efforts so far. Rectangle types hate feeling deprived.

The Rectangle type too, as I know from bitter experience, wants immediate results. If she can't lose one stone in two weeks, she can lose interest. But, as we all know, the best way—the only permanent way—is to lose weight solidly and steadily, re-learning our eating habits in the process. This can all sound too dull, and much too slow to the practical, active Rectangle.

So if you're feeling in desperate need of a culinary treat, keep off the chocolate or salami (once you start you find it very hard to stop). Instead, buy yourself some exotic and special fruit and keep it to eat and enjoy, all to yourself. A Rectangle friend of mine loves mangoes, and she says they're at their most delicious if eaten without any regard for manners or mess. So she saves herself the biggest and ripest mango, undresses and gets into her bath and sits there eating it to her utmost enjoyment, as the bright orange juice squelches over her face and runs down her front.

●By week three I was feeling great—had a bit of a platform over the weekend but then dropped 1.4 kg (3 lbs) so I was really pleased. My face looked thinner by this week. Exercising helped a great deal.●

Elyse

From talking to clients and from the evidence of my questionnaire I have found that chocolate cravings can be a real problem for some people, especially pre-menstrually. If you're in a stage of miserable craving, I think it is better to find a sensible way of dealing with this and I suggest you try a low-calorie chocolate drink (most of the leading brands are making one) as a safer substitute than demolishing a box of chocolates. This drink tastes chocolatey, feels naughty and is filling—really important for our sense of satisfaction. And I hope it will get rid of that awful sense of deprivation. But don't go getting addicted to this instead!

DAY FIFTEEN
Breakfast
40 g (1½ oz) unsweetened muesli, bran flakes, puffed wheat or any other unsweetened breakfast cereal, (with skimmed milk from daily allowance), cup tea or coffee.
Lunch
Quick pea soup (see recipe, on page 76) or 300 ml (½ pt) non-creamy packet soup (lentil/vegetable), one piece wholemeal bread, banana, cup of tea.
Supper
225 g (8 oz) white fish, grilled or steamed, green salad (as much as you like), low-cal dressing, either commercial brand or home-made (see recipe, on page 72), two-fruit salad, 1 tbsp low-fat natural yogurt.

DAY SIXTEEN
Breakfast
Two pieces wholemeal toast, low-fat spread from daily allowance, cup of tea or coffee.
Lunch
One hard-boiled egg, 25 g (1 oz) feta cheese chopped into large mixed salad (from permitted list), creamy low-cal dressing (see recipe, page 72), cup of tea.
Supper
Tandoori Chicken (see recipe, page 76), big salad or selection of vegetables (from permitted list),

Your exercise programme

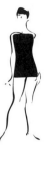

Increase your exercise repetitions as outlined in the box to the right. If you're finding your enthusiasm flag a little do try and keep up your exercise. There is a great deal of evidence that exercise is an anti-depressant. It is much better if you're feeling fed up and bored, hungry and rebellious, to go out and have an energetic game of squash, or a run. It keeps you from the fridge and improves your state of mind — and it burns calories.

I hope that those two floor exercises I gave you have improved your mobility in the waist and the muscle tone of your tummy. As I've said, nothing is going to give you a completely flat stomach, but strengthening the underlying muscles gives you the flattest profile possible for your shape.

EXERCISE REPETITIONS: WEEK THREE	
Waist Mobility Swing	10
Stomach and Waist Trimmer	5

baked apple cooked with two chopped dried apricots as stuffing, 1 tbsp frozen yogurt.

DAY SEVENTEEN
Breakfast
Either as Day 15 or Day 16.
Lunch
Bean and lentil salad (see recipe, page 75), 150 g (5 oz) low-fat fruit yogurt, cup of tea.
Supper
175 g (6 oz) fresh (grilled) or tinned tuna (in brine not oil), steamed vegetables (from permitted list), fresh fruit salad (from permitted list).

DAY EIGHTEEN
Breakfast
Either as Day 15 or Day 16.
Lunch
Mushroom omelette (see recipe, page 76), mixed salad, low-cal dressing (see recipe, page 72) or steamed vegetables, mango or any two fruits from permitted list.
Supper
Spaghetti with broccoli (see recipe, page 74), baked pepper salad (see recipe, page 77), one slice of wholemeal bread, banana split (1 tbsp iced vanilla yogurt instead of ice cream).

DAY NINETEEN
Breakfast
Either as Day 15 or Day 16.

Lunch
150 g (5 oz) cottage cheese mixed with chopped olives, radishes, spring onions, green salad, apple, cup of tea.
Supper
175 g (6 oz) rump steak grilled, steamed green vegetables (from permitted list), orange.

DAY TWENTY
Breakfast
Either as Day 15 or Day 16.
Lunch
Tabbouleh (see recipe, page 77) in wholemeal pitta bread, small bunch of grapes, cup of tea.
Supper
Salade Niçoise (see recipe, page 76), one slice of wholemeal bread, glass unsweetened fruit juice.

DAY TWENTY-ONE
Breakfast
Either as Day 15 or Day 16.
Lunch
Baked potato, 110 g (4 oz) baked beans, green salad, low-cal dressing (see recipe, page 72), cup of tea.
Supper
225 g (8 oz) white fish baked, steamed or grilled, tomato and onion salad, on bed of lettuce, low-cal dressing (see recipe, page 72), 50 g (2 oz) prunes, stewed, 1 tbsp low-fat natural yogurt.

RECTANGLE

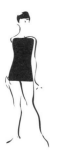

WEEK FOUR
Positive action: start at the top

JUST AS straight clothes suit Rectangle-type woman best, so do short, chic and angular hairstyles. Think of how much slimmer, chic-er and prettier Princess Diana looked when she had her long bob cut into her short, upswept style.

Unstructured, wavy, romantic hair which suits your curvy Pear and Hourglass friends can look untidy and frumpish on you. But if you have naturally curly hair, make sure it is cut in an angular style—either short and a bit spiky, or a jaw-length bob with a straight clubbed line at the back (see the illustration in the Triangle hairstyle section). Whatever your type of hair, do treat yourself to a good cut with a hair stylist who will take into consideration the weight and wave of your hair and the shape of your face.

If you want to change the colour of your hair, bear in mind that its natural tone is the one which suits your skin and eye colour best. Unless you are aiming for a dramatic look (dark-haired Madonna was never meant to be a blonde), keep within your natural colour range. Dramatic changes can look sensational when you're young (and can afford an expensive professional style—and its maintenance), but they are hardening and ageing to older skins.

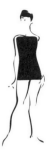

Professionally done high- and low-lights can be the most flattering way of adding zing to your hair without clashing with the rest of your colouring. But it can be expensive. I would always say that if you had to choose, a good cut is the priority. Your own hair colour, glossy and healthy on this diet, will then look as exciting as can be.

RECTANGLE

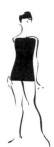

WEEK FOUR
Your diet

You are over the danger period of that third week. Although you may be disappointed that the scales do not register quite as much loss as you hoped I'm sure that by now you are feeling so much better—both slimmer and fitter—that you are quite happy to enter your fourth week. If Week Three had marked a plateau in your weight loss, then by the end of this fourth week I am pretty certain you will find you have lost *more* than you hoped. Friends will certainly be noticing the effects in your face.

DAY TWENTY-TWO
Breakfast
40 g (1½ oz) unsweetened muesli, bran flakes, puffed wheat or any other unsweetened breakfast cereal, (with skimmed milk from daily allowance), cup of tea or coffee.
Lunch
100 g (4 oz) peeled prawns, large mixed salad, creamy low-cal dressing (see recipe, page 72), orange, cup of tea.
Supper
Ratatouille (see recipe, page 74) with 50 g (2 oz) rice (dry weight, preferably brown) boiled, ginger banana (see recipe, page 79).

•Everyone I know is impressed by my weight-loss and wants to try the diet. At the start of the diet I told Bel I am not going to be fat and 40. When I hit 40 in August, thanks to the diet, "Life Begins At 40" will apply to me.•

Diane

DAY TWENTY-THREE
Breakfast
Two pieces of wholemeal toast, low-fat spread from daily allowance, cup of tea or coffee.
Lunch
100 g (4 oz) cottage cheese, apple and orange chopped in, cup of tea.
Supper
175 g (6 oz) chicken breast, rubbed with 1 tsp olive oil and herbs, grilled, selection of vegetables (from permitted list), baked apple cooked with two dried apricots as stuffing, 1 tbsp low-fat natural yogurt.

DAY TWENTY-FOUR
Breakfast
Either as Day 22 or Day 23.
Lunch
300 ml (½ pt) any non-creamy packet soup or homemade vegetable soup (see recipe, page 75), one piece of wholemeal bread/toast, banana, cup of tea.
Supper
200 g (7 oz) smoked haddock, steamed or poached in skimmed milk (from daily allowance) and water, two to more vegetables (from permitted list), one piece of fruit cut into 150 g (5 oz) low-fat natural yogurt.

DAY TWENTY-FIVE
Breakfast
Either as Day 22 or Day 23.
Lunch
Spanish omelette (see recipe, page 76), green salad, low-cal dressing (see recipe, page 72), one piece of fruit (from permitted list).
Supper
Chick pea curry (see recipe, page 74), 25 g (1 oz) rice (dry weight, preferably brown) boiled, banana split with 1 tbsp frozen natural yogurt instead of ice cream.

RECTANGLE

Celebration treat:
buy something RED

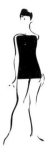

You've got there. Four weeks of a new way of eating and an exercise programme both of which are tailor-made for your body type and I hope you are really feeling more energetic, more attractive, more *you*. To celebrate, I would like to suggest that you go and buy yourself something red. It can be anything from a red scarf or handkerchief to red earrings, a jersey or—if you're feeling really triumphant—a red dress.

But remember, there are many shades of red. There are blue reds and orange reds; clear bright reds or muted, blended reds; light or deep reds. Before buying yourself your red treat, hold it under your chin to check it is a flattering red for *you*. The right red will give you a healthy glow, and your skin, hair and eyes will look more vibrant. The wrong red will make you pale and washed out. Any blemishes and dark shadows on your face are emphasized by the wrong colours.

Red is a marvellous colour. It lifts the spirits. It makes a definite statement; not 'poor little over-weight mousy me, please let me pass by, unseen in the crowd', but rather, 'I AM FULL OF LIFE! I AM CONFIDENT, I AM HAPPY, LOOK AT ME!'

DAY TWENTY-SIX

Breakfast
Either as Day 22 or Day 23.

Lunch
100 g (4 oz) cottage cheese, baked pepper and anchovy (see recipe, page 77), one piece of fruit, cup of tea.

Supper
Mixed grill of two back rashers bacon (all fat trimmed off), one lamb's kidney, two small low-fat sausages, tomatoes, mushrooms (all grilled, not fried), green side salad, low-cal dressing (see recipe, page 72), 150 g (5 oz) low-fat natural yogurt, chopped apple, few raisins.

DAY TWENTY-SEVEN

Breakfast
Either as Day 22 or Day 23.

Lunch
Baked potato, 1 tbsp hummus, mixed salad, low-cal dressing (see recipe, page 72), 150 g (5 oz) low-fat fruit yogurt, cup of tea.

Supper
Kyoto Trout Salad (see recipe, page 75), stewed prunes and apricots (two of each), 1 tbsp frozen natural yogurt.

DAY TWENTY-EIGHT

Breakfast
Either as Day 22 or Day 23.

Your exercise programme

You can now increase the repetitions of your waist exercises as outlined in the box below. I hope that by now you have also established a routine of swimming, running, aerobic sports, cycling or vigorous exercise class or video and are really seeing the benefits in toned-up muscles, extra weight loss and improved circulation and spirits. You should be able to work out a pattern of exercise which is not too ambitious and will be easy and pleasurable to follow in the long term. Here's to a fitter, happier you!

EXERCISE REPETITIONS: WEEK FOUR	
Waist Mobility Swing	12
Stomach and Waist Trimmer	6

Lunch
Three fruits (from permitted list) made into fruit salad with 150g (5 oz) low-fat natural yogurt or 75 g (3 oz) fromage frais (8% fat), cup of tea.

Supper
Quarter of chicken, grilled or dry roasted, large mixed salad, low-cal dressing (see recipe, page 72), one piece of fruit.

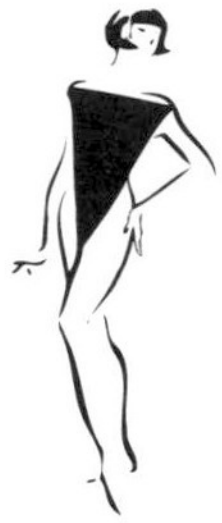

TRIANGLE

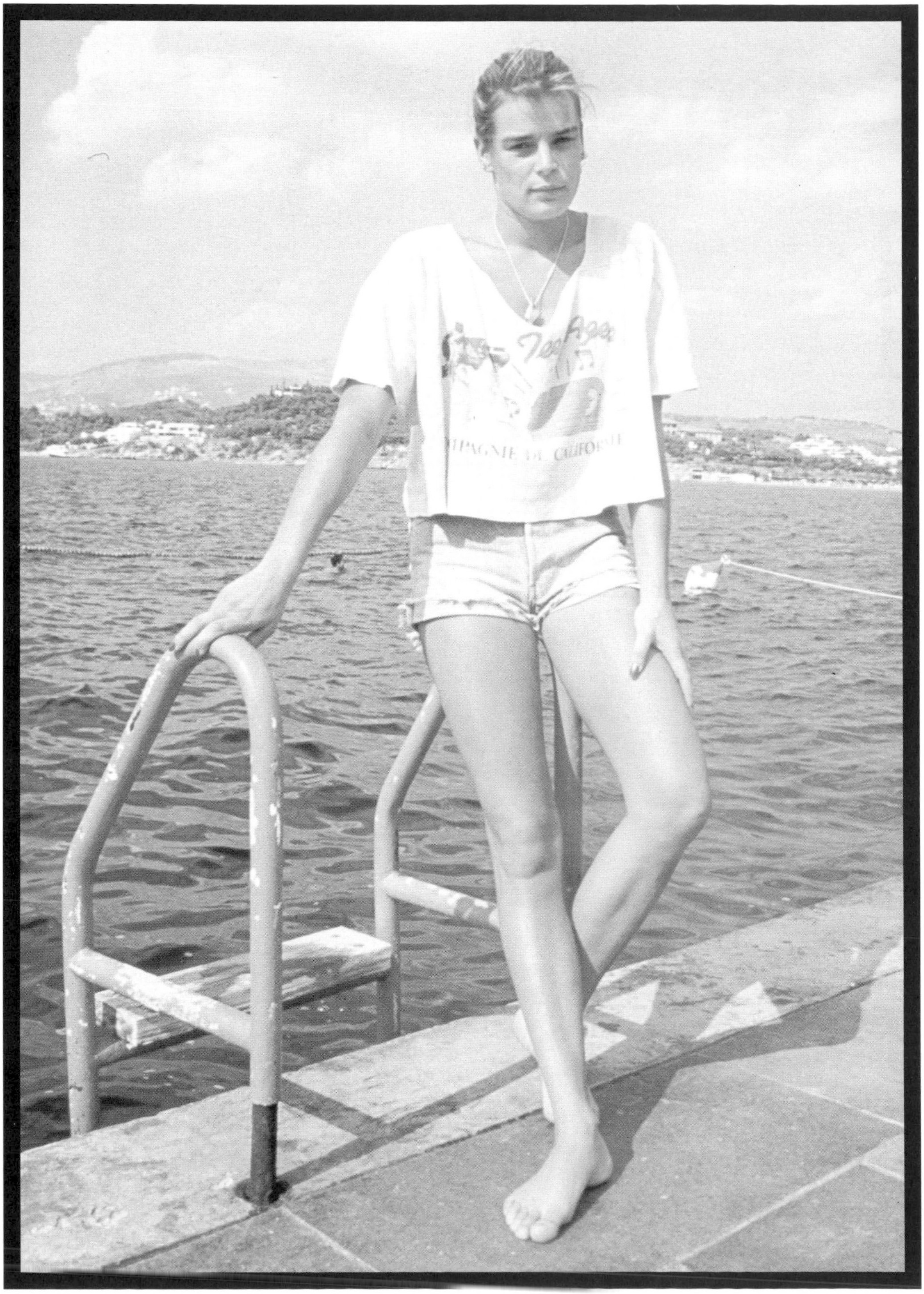

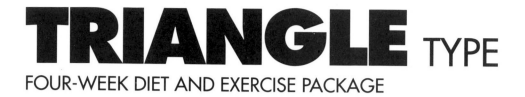

TRIANGLE TYPE

FOUR-WEEK DIET AND EXERCISE PACKAGE

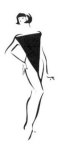

THIS IS a four-week package of diet menus and exercise programme tailor-made for your body type and metabolism. A team of volunteer dieters tested this diet and exercise programme for six weeks and some for three months or more. Their experiences and comments went into improving it for you.

With each week, my volunteer dieters and I found it was very encouraging to have a treat, or 'positive action', to lift our spirits and keep us going for the next week. As you read through the package you will see what I mean.

Individual characteristics

The Triangle type is likely to have been slim as a teenager, athletic, and with a big appetite. In adulthood, the demands of a family and career can mean she does less exercise, eats the wrong things at wrong times, still has an unrestrained appetite and she can then start putting on weight. Although the Triangle type rarely puts on a lot of weight, she is very organized and disciplined and when she decides to do something about her shape she works out a routine and readily sticks to it.

She tends to be an early riser whose energy levels are at their best in the morning. Consequently, her metabolism deals best with a diet which gives her a hearty breakfast, and a main meal at lunchtime with only a light evening meal. To get through the latter part of the day, when the Triangle-type's energy is running down, this diet allows a small metabolic-boosting snack in the afternoon.

This type positively *needs* regular, energetic exercise and can get depressed if she isn't doing any. In our questionnaire, 75 per cent of our Triangle types said they recognized that they needed to exercise *and* diet if they were to lose weight—and it was energetic exercise which they favoured—a much higher proportion than the other body types (for instance, only 30 per cent of the Pear types thought exercise important).

The Triangle type is at her best when doing regular aerobic exercise, ie exercise which raises the heart rate like aerobics, speed swimming, jogging, bicycling. She tends to be physically well co-ordinated and energetic dancing, like jazz, or tap, appeals to her too.

Princess Stephanie of Monaco is an archetypal Triangle of the sporty type—her naturally broad shoulders are enhanced by exercise. More petite versions of this shape are Mia Farrow, Annie Lennox and Jackie Onassis. Unlike the Rectangle, this body type has hips which are distinctly narrower than her shoulders. Hips and legs are lean and straight. This is a shape many top sportswomen share.

The Triangle looks really marvellous in sporty clothes like these, but more formal wear has to be crisp and tailored. Evening wear is the most difficult area of dress for Princess Stephanie and all Triangle types. Frills, flounces, cinched waists and full skirts should always be avoided in favour of simple geometric lines—like a sheath dress in a rich, crisp fabric; silk gaberdine, lamé, or beaded and sequinned work on a strong base fabric. Although this shape is the most masculine of our body types, it is the Triangle-type woman who can most easily look chic and elegant, expressing her femininity not through frills but with well-cut clothes which follow her tapering body line.

TRIANGLE

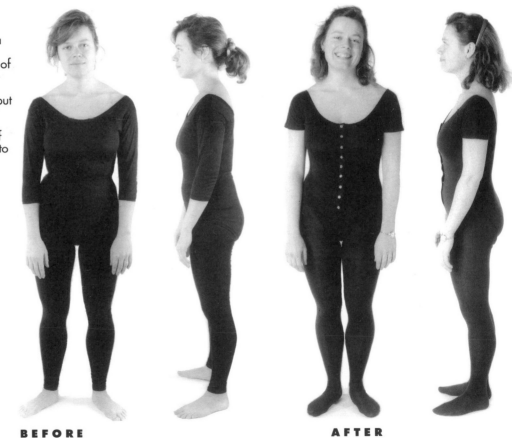

TRIANGLE-TYPE WEIGHT AND MEASUREMENTS BEFORE DIETING, AND SIX WEEKS LATER

NAME	WEIGHT (kg/st & lbs) BEFORE	WEIGHT (kg/st & lbs) AFTER	MEASUREMENTS (cms/ins) BEFORE BUST	BEFORE WAIST	HIPS	AFTER BUST	AFTER WAIST	HIPS
Liz	54/8 8	51/8 2	87.5/35	71/28½	90.5/36¼	87.5/35	69/27½	90/36
Rita	50.5/8 0	46/7 5	90/36	73/29¼	87.5/35	87.5/35	70/28	85/34
Judith	54/8 8	51/8 1	85/34	66/26½	91/36½	81/32½	62/24¾	85/34
Nita	66/10 7	62/9 12	91/36½	72.5/29	96/38½	90/36	67.5/27	87.5/35
Betty	60/9 8	57/9 1	95/38	72.5/29	94/37½	89/35½	72.5/29	92.5/37
Sally	75/11 13	70/11 10	107.5/43	81/32½	102.5/41	101/40½	70.5/28¼	92.5/37
Ros	64/10 3	61/9 10	90/36	70/28	95/38	90/36	70/28	85/34

None of the Triangle-type volunteers had a lot of weight to lose as this type of woman is hormonally less predisposed to put on weight (see Science section, page 16) and, if she does, tends to do something about it pretty quickly.

BEFORE

AFTER

With a weight loss of 3 kg (7 lbs) in six weeks, our volunteer above is slimmer on her upper chest, spare tyre and tummy, narrowing her body profile. Although her bust and waist measurements remained the same, she lost a dramatic 10 cms (4 ins) off her upper hips, again re-emphasizing the triangular shape.

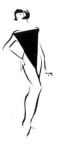

TRIANGLE-TYPE DIETERS' WEIGHT LOSS OVER SIX WEEKS (kgs/lbs)

NAME	WEEK:	1	2	3	4	5	6	TOTAL WEIGHT LOSS
Liz		0.9/2	0.5/1	0.9/2	0.5/1	0/0	0/0	−2.7/6
Rita		1.8/4	0.5/1	0/0	0.5/1	0/0	1.4/3	−4/9
Judith		0/0	0.5/1	0/0	+0.5/1	0/0	3.1/7	−3.1/7
Nita		1.4/3	0.9/2	1.8/4	0/0	0/0	0/0	−4/9
Betty		1.4/3	0.5/1	0/0	0/0	0/0	1.4/3	−3.1/7
Sally		1.4/3	1.8/4	0.5/1	0.5/1	0/0	1.4/3	−5.5/12
Ros		1.4/3	1.8/4	0.25/ ½	0.25/½	0/0	+0.5/1	−3.1/7

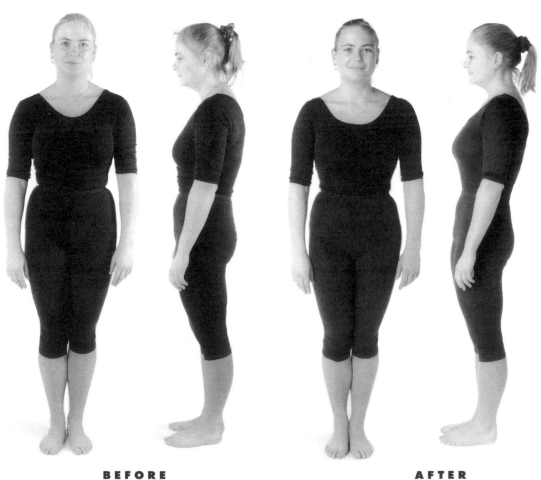

BEFORE

AFTER

Our volunteer above felt she'd put on weight because she had been unable to get to the gym regularly for work-outs. She therefore combined work-outs with the Triangle-type diet to lose 5.5 kg (12 lbs) in six weeks – virtually reaching her ideal weight in that time. Weight has come off most dramatically from her waist (10 cms

[4¼ ins]) and upper hips (10 cms [4 ins]), as well as her upper chest, spare tyre and tummy.

This volunteer's weight loss emphasized her broad-shouldered, narrow-hipped shape, ie she became more triangular in shape. Her body profile is narrower and her face is also slimmer and more defined.

TRIANGLE

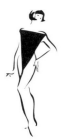

WEEK ONE
Positive action: enhance your style

AS YOU'VE already seen, we don't all share the same body shape and an outfit that looks fantastic on one person can look dreadful on somebody else. And this is not just a matter of slenderness. Wearing clothes which suit your body shape, rather than hiding your good points and drawing attention to your bad, can give you the appearance of having *lost 3 kg (7 lbs)* before you even begin your diet.

The Triangle type has broader shoulders than hips and more of a marked waist than the Rectangle. She falls into two basic types, the small boned, boyish figure like Mia Farrow and Annie Lennox who probably rarely, if ever, puts on weight and the more muscular, athletic looking type, like Princess Stephanie of Monaco, Jamie Lee Curtis, Grace Jones and Angelica Huston, who can get heavy in the upper torso area, but keeps her inverted triangle shape with straight hips and lean lower legs. When thin, this type is the classic fashion model shape with coat-hanger shoulders, next-to-nothing-hips and long slim legs.

The basic principle of style is that you wear clothes which have the same or similar line to your body line. So, for the Triangle, whatever your size, keep everything angled and sharp. Your jackets and tops should have straight, angular shoulders and should taper from shoulder to waist. Skirts and trousers similarly should be narrow, tapering into the hem or ankle. Any gathers can make you look heavy or dowdy. The Triangle type often has good athletic legs and looks best in short skirts, jeans or leggings (but they must be made of a substantial fabric which keeps its lean shape and doesn't bag or wrinkle).

Some women with this body type try to counteract their broad-shouldered look by wearing flimsy, ultra 'feminine' clothes—think of Diane Keaton (a Triangle type) in *Annie Hall*. Those soft, drifty clothes (which would have looked more at home on an Hourglass, like Julia Roberts) on the angular Diane make her look a bit like Little Orphan Annie, rather gawky and fey.

This suited the character very well in the film, but for you, wanting to be taken seriously in the real world, it can be a counter-productive look. Your femininity is best expressed with clothes that have simple geometric lines, certainly angled to the waist if you like, but it's better to avoid soft fabrics, gathers and bows. It is always best to follow the line of your body and you—like the Rectangle—need angular, rather than curvy clothes, to look your best—and slimmest.

Fabrics need to be close woven and crisp—too soft and crumpled, like linen, and you can look a mess. Gaberdines, wool, crisp cottons and heavy silk all look smart and sharp enough. Shiny materials like leather and lamé also suit your type.

All details on clothing and accessories need to be angular rather than curvy; lapels, jacket edges, belt buckles, shoes and handbags. (Beware scoop necklines, which can make you look very broad and heavy in the shoulder.)

If you are very overweight
Although the Triangle body type is not often heavily overweight, you may feel that these general style pointers are a bit extreme for your larger shape and so here are some possible modifications.

However heavy you get, you will retain slim lower legs and be relatively narrow in the lower hips. Show off your legs with knee-length narrow skirts—anything shorter will emphasize your top-heaviness. If you really feel you want a skirt with a bit more ease then straight pleats will suit you, but try to keep the lower profile narrow. Never wear anything gathered and waisted, it will only make you look much bulkier and frumpy. Your shape looks excellent in narrow legged trousers with a straight tunic or jacket—the Principal Boy look suits you well.

If you're young or can get away with informal dressing, good quality leggings (ones which don't sag and bag) with a crisp man's shirt or good quality straight top or large jersey with a straight line, like a fisherman's rib, can look good. Keep your shoulder line straight with good shoulder pads.

Your extra weight is predominantly on your tummy, spare tyre, bust and shoulders and so you

TRIANGLE

may feel that a jacket that is straight, rather than tapering to the waist, is more flattering.

Good accessories become all the more necessary for the overweight woman who wants to dress well. A good square handbag, chisel-toed shoes and an important piece of geometric jewellery (see section overleaf) can all add crispness and authority to your look.

TRIANGLE

TRIANGLE

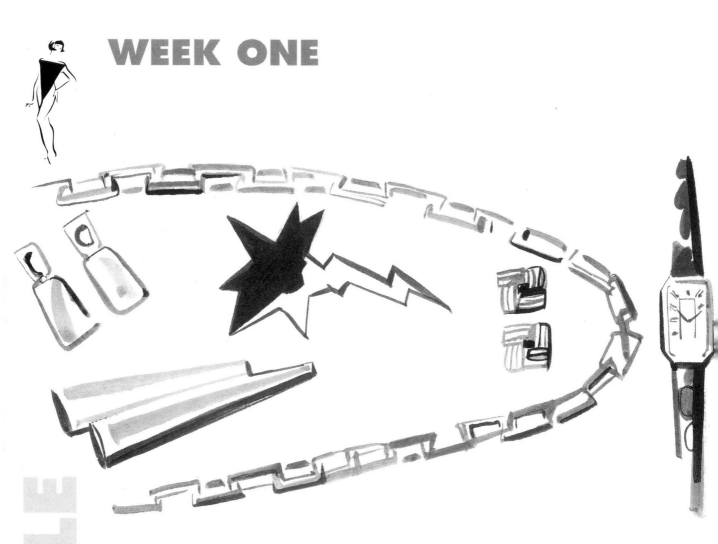

Jewellery

Jewellery for the Triangle type follows the same line as her body and her clothes. Keep detail angular at all times. Chain links should be flat rather than curvy, necklaces with round beads are not becoming.

Brooches and earrings look better if they are unfussy and geometric. Squares, diamond-shapes, rectangles, triangles and variations of these, look really classy on this type—regardless of the cost of the piece—whereas curved shapes, however expensive the jewellery, can look just cheap.

But remember, scale is as important in jewellery as it is in clothes. It has to be in the right size for you. If you are large boned (as a rough guide if your wrist measures 16.5cms [6½ins] or more) then your jewellery pieces ought to be large and important. If you are medium (14 to 16.5cms [5½ to 6½ins]) to

small boned (less than 14cms [5½ins]) then make sure your jewellery is more delicate and on a smaller scale so that it doesn't overwhelm you.

Watches for the Triangle type are better if their faces are square or rectangular. Again, scale is important; if you are large boned you may find some of the more elegant men's watches suit you best. Keep all detail unfussy and everything you wear should have clean sharp lines. This way every piece of clothing and accessory will look classy, and you much more chic.

So, as your first positive action, make yourself feel better and look slimmer in the right clothes and accessories for your shape. Then, confidence boosted by your new appearance, start on the first week of your tailor-made diet and exercise plan and begin to lose *real* pounds of weight.

Starting your diet

This is a low-fat diet. With a reduced fat, reduced sugar and increased fibre intake, this diet takes into account the latest findings on healthy nutrition. There is a good deal of evidence though that the Triangle type needs more protein than the other body types and should not have too many dairy products.

With your regular aerobic exercise routine you will increase your metabolic rate and therefore are allowed a few more calories in your diet than the more sedentary types.

In response to your active morning metabolism, the most efficient diet for this type is a protein breakfast, substantial lunch, late-afternoon snack and light supper. Such a breakfast may be difficult to fit in to a busy life but will help keep your energy levels high and keep your metabolism burning through the day.

A substantial lunch too can cause problems unless you are working at home or eating in restaurants or canteens most days. A packed lunch, however, with a piece of cold chicken for instance, wholemeal roll, raw carrots, or other salad vegetables, will do very well. No snacking allowed, apart from the permitted afternoon snack.

The menus which follow are for those of you who like a structured diet. For the rest, they are suggestions for meals based on the basic principles of your body-type diet of lean protein (lots of fish, lean meat, eggs), unrefined carbohydrates (like baked potato, wholemeal bread, brown rice), with almost limitless salad and vegetables, and generous amounts of fruit.

You can switch meals around from day to day—or repeat easy or favourite ones—as long as you have lunches at lunchtime and suppers in the evening. Useful, though not ideal, if you are too busy, or disinclined to cook, are the ready-made, low-calorie frozen meals. You may substitute these for your main meal but add a salad or vegetables.

This diet does not allow for alcohol. There are two main reasons for this: alcohol represents empty calories and I would rather you got food value for your extra calories in the shape of an extra piece of fruit, or another helping of salad or vegetables—or even a slightly larger helping of protein: fish or eggs or chicken. But most importantly, alcohol undermines our self-control—and can be to addictive. Once we've had one drink it's much easier to have another, and then our resolve goes and we're eating anything that comes our way.

DAILY ALLOWANCE

300 ml (½ pt) skimmed milk
15 g (½ oz) low-fat spread

Beverages: try to keep your intake of tea/coffee to two cups a day, but drink plenty of water and have as many cups of herb tea as you like

Unlimited vegetables (preferably raw, otherwise boiled/steamed):

asparagus	aubergine	bean sprouts	beetroot
broccoli	brussel sprouts	cabbage	carrots
cauliflower	celery	chard	chicory
courgettes	cucumbers	French beans	endive
escarole	green/red pepper	kale	lettuce
mange-tout peas	mushrooms	okra	onions
parsley	radishes	runner beans	spinach
spring greens	tomatoes	turnips	watercress

SB: Permitted fruits where indicated (no smacking!):

apple	apricot	handful blackberries	grapefruit
kiwi	nectarine	orange	peach
pear	plum	tangerine	slice watermelon

WEEK ONE

It's much easier and generally more efficient if you can cut out alcohol for the duration of your diet. Many women find that they can lose weight just by doing this, so unaware were they of how many extra calories they were consuming every day in liquid form. However, I am aware that for some women this is an impossibility and if it is the difference between going on the diet or not, obviously I would rather you follow the dieting guidelines and limit your alcohol to one drink a day, preferably with your meal.

For vegetarians there are recipes for main meal substitutions in the recipe supplement on pages 72–9.

This diet should not only help the Triangle type to lose weight but to be healthier, look better and feel great.

DAY ONE

Breakfast
Two eggs, scrambled or any style (OR 100 g (4 oz) kipper fillet grilled OR two pieces back bacon, fat removed, grilled OR half 120 g (4 oz) tin sardines in brine, drained) on one slice of wholemeal toast, low-fat spread from daily allowance, cup tea or coffee.

'Eating a large breakfast or lunch for my main meal kept my energy level high during the day when I most needed it. I felt very active and craved exercise for that all-over 'good feeling'. It's also good to know that the calories got burned up too.'

Rita

Lunch
225 g (8 oz) white fish, grilled or steamed, two small boiled potatoes, large green salad (from permitted vegetables), low-cal dressing, either commercial brand or home-made (see recipe, page 72), two-fruit salad.

Late-afternoon snack
Two pieces of crispbread spread with 25 g (1 oz) anchovy paste, sandwich spread, vegetable pâté or any low-fat pâté, sliced cucumber on top.

Supper
300ml (½ pt) any non-creamy packet soup or homemade vegetable soup (see recipe, page 75), one slice of wholemeal bread/toast.

DAY TWO

Breakfast
Same as above.

Lunch
Spaghetti with broccoli (see recipe, page 74), sliced tomato and onion salad with low-cal dressing (see recipe, page 72), one slice of wholemeal bread, banana split (1 tbsp iced vanilla yogurt instead of ice cream).

Late-afternoon snack
25 g (1 oz) packet savoury popcorn.

Supper
Half avocado, 50 g (2 oz) prawns, green salad, low-cal dressing (see recipe, page 72).

DAY THREE

Breakfast
Same as above.

Lunch
Tandoori chicken (see recipe, page 76), selection of vegetables (from permitted list), baked apple cooked with two dried apricots as stuffing, 1 tbsp low-fat natural yogurt.

Late-afternoon snack
Large banana.

Supper
Red cabbage, apple & hazelnut salad (see recipe, page 77).

TRIANGLE

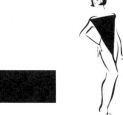

DAY FOUR
Breakfast
Same as above but *not* eggs.
Lunch
Baked potato, 110 g (4 oz) baked beans, two back rashers bacon, trimmed and grilled, low-cal coleslaw or homemade with creamy low-cal dressing (see recipe, page 72).
Late-afternoon snack
50 g (2 oz) olives, raw carrot, celery sticks, 1 tbsp hummus.
Supper
One poached egg on spinach (frozen or fresh, any amount), one wholemeal roll or slice of bread.

DAY FIVE
Breakfast
Same as above.
Lunch
Stir-fry beef with mange-tout (see recipe, page 75), green vegetables (from permitted list), boiled or steamed, orange.
Late-afternoon snack
Two crispbreads spread with 25 g (1 oz) fish paste, or low-fat pâté, sliced cucumber on top.
Supper
Baked pepper salad (see recipe, page 77), one wholemeal roll.

DAY SIX
Breakfast
Same as above.
Lunch
175 g (6 oz) fresh (grilled) or tinned tuna (in brine not oil), steamed vegetables (from permitted list), 40 g (1½ oz) rice (dried weight, preferably brown) boiled, two-fruit salad.
Late-afternoon snack
Cereal bar (under 100 cals).
Supper
Tabbouleh (see recipe, page 77) in wholemeal pitta bread.

'I'm a real morning person, an early riser, and I loathe eating a big meal in the evening because it then sits heavily on me all evening and I find I sleep less well.

There's something really interesting about this different body type metabolism. I know that the pattern of my eating and exercising is naturally quite opposite to that of my Pear-shape sister. At last a diet which takes these important differences into consideration. It *is* a breakthrough!'

Liz

DAY SEVEN
Breakfast
Same as above.
Lunch
Quarter chicken, roasted/grilled, one wholemeal roll or slice of bread, large mixed salad (from permitted list), low-cal dressing (see recipe, page 72), ginger banana (see recipe, page 79)
Late-afternon snack
Apple and orange.
Supper
Quick pea soup (see recipe, page 76), one slice of wholemeal bread.

TRIANGLE

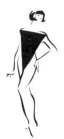

WEEK ONE
Your exercise programme

This body type thrives on exercise—vigorous, aerobic exercise. I suggest that, together with your dieting regime, you do *at least* three periods of half an hour, or more, solid aerobic exercise each week. This can take the form of aerobics, speed swimming, jazz, tap or other modern dance, running, jogging, bicycling. Some of you probably exercise daily already, ideally in the mornings.

The most vigorous exercise burns up 10 calories a minute, which represents 300 calories for half an hour's exercise. But more than the obvious energy-burning advantage of exercise, aerobic exercise like this markedly boosts the metabolism for quite a few hours after you have stopped. It also has the effect for women with this body shape of increasing the general feeling of well-being and fitness.

Triangle types can be obsessional and run some risk of overdoing their exercise routines. If you feel you are getting tired and run down, or you're beginning to injure muscles and sprain joints, you must be careful to give your body time to recover.

Although I know your body type tends to prefer active exercise and can find floor exercises rather boring I have suggested these three floor exercises as strengtheners and toners of tummy muscles, and arm, chest, and midriff. But if you're already into a good mixed regime of exercise you may not need to add them to your programme. Good Luck.

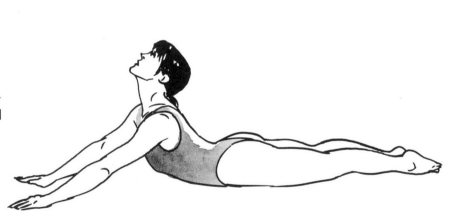

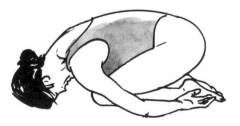

Modified cat stretch

1 Lie flat on the floor face down, legs together and stretched out behind you in a straight line. Keep your palms flat on the floor under your shoulders.

2 Push down on your hands as you raise your head and upper torso. Curl your head and spine up and backwards as far as you can go, with your arms straight, your shoulders down and still keeping your hips on the floor.

3 Stretch back that little extra inch. *Hold the position while you count to ten.*

4 Then very slowly, lower yourself to the floor.

5 *Repeat this part of the exercise five times.*

6 Rise to a kneeling position, sitting on your feet. Tuck your head between your knees and round your shoulders to form a ball.

7 Slip your arms down to lie loosely alongside your legs.

8 Relax.

Stomach clincher

1 Sit on the floor, legs wide apart and arms straight out at your sides at shoulder level.
2 Slowly bend forward and twist, trying to touch your right knee with your forehead. Don't worry if you can't do this at the first attempt—as you become fitter you will get closer and closer. At the same time, slowly slide your left hand down your right leg, reaching as far towards (or beyond) your foot as you can. Stretch your right arm out behind you.
3 Return slowly to the starting position and repeat, taking your forehead to touch the left leg.
REPEAT WHOLE EXERCISE FIVE TIMES.

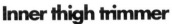

Inner thigh trimmer

Although you'll feel this exercise working primarily on the muscles of the inner thigh (where your type can put on weight), it will also help shape and firm up your waist and stomach.

1 Lie on your back on the floor in front of a sturdy chair.
2 Straighten your legs and grip the outside edge of the two front legs of the chair with your feet. Place your arms by your sides.
3 Push as hard as you can against the chair legs, as if you were trying to close your legs.
4 At the same time, lift your head and shoulders, but try to keep your shoulders relaxed, and look at your toes.
5 *Hold this position for a count of 30 (you may find you need to build up to this count over a few days).*
6 Relax.
REPEAT EXERCISE TWO TIMES.

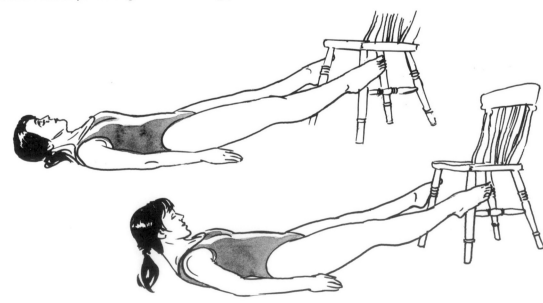

TRIANGLE

59

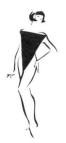

WEEK TWO
Positive action: instant healthy glow

GO AND buy yourself a blusher. Nothing lifts the contours of a face and the colour of a complexion more immediately and naturally than blusher. Buy a powder in a neutral rosy tone and apply it as shown in the illustration below.

1 Brush blush along the cheekbone, starting on a level with the outer edge of your iris and feathering it upwards and outwards as far as the hairline at the top of your ear.

2 You might like also to add the slightest touch of colour to your temples and chin.

3 Blend the edges with a soft powder brush. Never have definite lines in any make-up you apply.

Many women say to me that they don't use make-up and it usually means they are not confident about using it and don't like a made-up look. My answer is that from our mid-twenties onwards our colouring tends to fade and the definition of our features softens with age. I never advocate a stagey effect, but do point out that if you are in business, well-applied make-up gives your features greater definition and adds more authority to your whole image.

If you still feel reluctant or lacking in competence, try using just your new blusher and a soft neutral lipstick. This should make your complexion brighter, your eyes more intense in colour and your face more contoured.

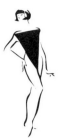

Subtly applied eye make-up needs a bit more technique and practice. But it is eye make-up which many fair-skinned, light-eyelashed women particularly feel they need. In my classes, even the most tentative women manage a professional job after experimenting for half an hour. Without being able to advise you personally, taking into account your individual colouring and shape of eye, I can only give the following steps as a general pointer.

Triangle types can put on weight on their faces and shoulders so you may well be noticing by now that your first week's dieting has begun to reveal more marked cheekbones and a cleaner jawline—and a longer, slimmer neck. Certainly, on this diet your skin will improve, although you may find that during the first week it's a bit spotty as you clear some of the toxins out of your system.

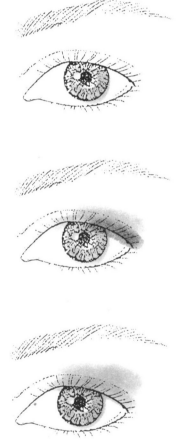

1 Highlighter: using an eyeshadow sponge, apply a light, neutral colour on the whole area of your upper eye from eyelid to brow.

2 Lid: apply a light to medium colour just on the lid (a taupe or soft olive suit most people), blending with a small brush.

3 Orbital bone: apply a darker colour along the upper eye-socket crease, blending it onto the lid at the outer corner of the eye. Blend all the colours with a soft brush. The end result must look like a wash of colour over your lid, getting darker towards the socket and the outside edge. No stripes or hard edges please.

4 Mascara: finish off the look with a couple of coats of brown mascara on the upper lashes, and one coat on the lower.

TRIANGLE

61

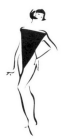

WEEK TWO
Your diet

DAY EIGHT

Breakfast

Two eggs, scrambled or any style (OR 100 g (4 oz) kipper fillet grilled OR half 120 g (4 oz) tin sardines in brine) on one slice of wholemeal toast, low-fat spread from daily allowance, cup of tea or coffee.

Lunch

Salade Niçoise (see recipe, page 76), one wholemeal roll, mango, paw paw, or two pieces of fruit from permitted list.

Late-afternoon snack

25 g (1 oz) packet savoury popcorn.

Supper

Ratatouille (see recipe, page 74).

DAY NINE

Breakfast

Same as above.

Lunch

Kyoto trout salad (see recipe, page 75), piece of wholemeal bread, low-fat spread from daily allowance, 50 g (2 oz) prunes, stewed.

Late-afternoon snack

25 g (1 oz) packet twiglets, OR two crispbreads spread with marmite.

Supper

Green salad with four pecan nuts, low-cal dressing (see recipe, page 72).

DAY TEN

Breakfast

Same as above, but *not* eggs.

Lunch

Spanish omelette (see recipe, page 76), one slice of wholemeal bread, large salad (from permitted list), 150 g (5 oz) low-fat fruit yogurt.

Late-afternoon snack

Large banana.

Supper

225 g (8 oz) baked beans on one slice of wholemeal toast.

DAY ELEVEN

Breakfast

Same as above.

Lunch

Chick pea curry (see recipe, page 74), 50 g (2 oz) rice (dried weight, preferably brown) boiled, steamed broccoli, carrots, or any other vegetables from permitted list, one slice of fruit.

Late-afternoon snack

Cereal bar (under 100 cals).

Supper

Stuffed tomatoes (see recipe, page 73), one piece of crispbread

DAY TWELVE

Breakfast

Same as above.

Lunch

Stir-fry chicken and vegetables (see recipe, page 72), 210 g (8 oz) can of any fruit in own juice.

Late-afternoon snack

Two pieces of crispbread spread with 25 g (1 oz) low-fat pâté, sliced cucumber on top.

Supper

Baked pepper and anchovy (see recipe, page 77), one wholemeal roll.

DAY THIRTEEN

Breakfast

Same as above.

Lunch

200 g (7 oz) white fish (grilled, steamed or baked), broccoli, courgettes, or any other vegetables (from permitted list), one wholemeal roll, stewed prunes and apricots (two of each).

Late-afternoon snack

Orange and apple.

Supper

Small baked potato, 1 dessertsp hummus, green side salad.

TRIANGLE

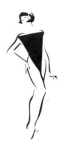

'Your description fits me remarkably well. I am a Triangle but become more rectangular when I put on weight. As you say, my best time of the day is morning and I get up at 6 o'clock in order to use that efficiently. I need a reasonable breakfast and lunch to keep me going. I suffer if I don't exercise. As a teenager I swam and danced and now, even though I work 60 hours a week sometimes and have two small children, I will always find time for my advanced ballet class which I love.'

Betty

DAY FOURTEEN

Breakfast
Same as above.

Lunch
Vegetable casserole (see recipe, page 73), 50 g (2 oz) rice (dried weight, preferably brown) boiled, green salad (from permitted list), low-cal dressing (see recipe, page 72), baked apple with two chopped dates as stuffing, 1 tbsp fromage frais (8% fat).

Late-afternoon snack
One slice of wholemeal toast spread with fish paste or low-fat pâté.

Supper
Half avocado, 50 g (2 oz) prawns, green salad (from permitted list), low-cal dressing (see recipe, page 72).

Your exercise programme

Maintain your daily exercise programme as outlined in the box below.

I hope that you're feeling fitter and lighter now and are beginning to see the positive benefits in hard exercise. If you're unused to it, it may take some self-discipline to get yourself going on a regime but you, of all the body shapes, are able to set yourself a goal and really stick with it. This is one of the positive elements in your natural competitiveness. If getting to the gym or to aerobics classes is difficult you may feel like borrowing one of the more demanding aerobics videos and doing the programme at home.

EXERCISE REPETITIONS: WEEK TWO	
Modified Cat Stretch	5
Stomach Clincher	6
Inner Thigh Trimmer	3

TRIANGLE

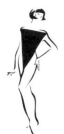

WEEK THREE
Positive action: good foundations

YOU ARE due for a reward for having got this far and lost those first pounds—some of you may be as much as 3 kg (7 lbs) lighter by this point, others more like 1.8–2.3 kg (4–5 lbs). Whatever weight you have lost, you will notice a flattening of the bulges—particularly probably your tummy. You may well feel like treating yourself to an indulgence that does not involve food. I suggest a glamorous piece of underwear which will make you feel pampered and proud of your increasingly fit body.

Women with straight hips are more flattered by sporty underwear and you can't get away with anything frilly. That doesn't mean you can't buy sexy underwear—sexy for you means those sporty, high-cut knickers, or short boxers, or triangular bikinis. French knickers are best left to the curvy hipped women. If you want lace, make sure it's not flimsy or frilly. Satin looks good on you but again you'll find it much more becoming to keep necklines and leg lines angular rather than curved.

A pretty underwired satin bra will give you good support, or you may prefer the crossed-back sporty bra. A satin all-in-one can be very flattering, but make sure any lace insets are angular and made of good quality lace. Spoil yourself.

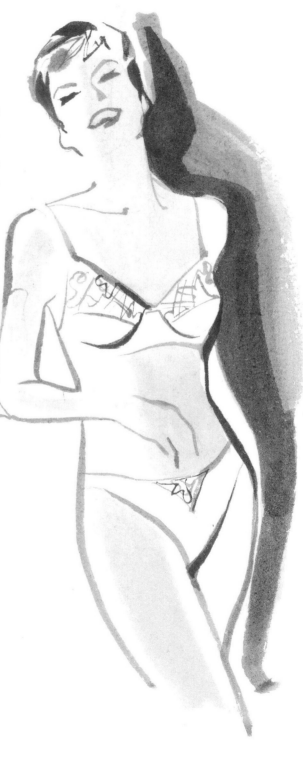

TRIANGLE

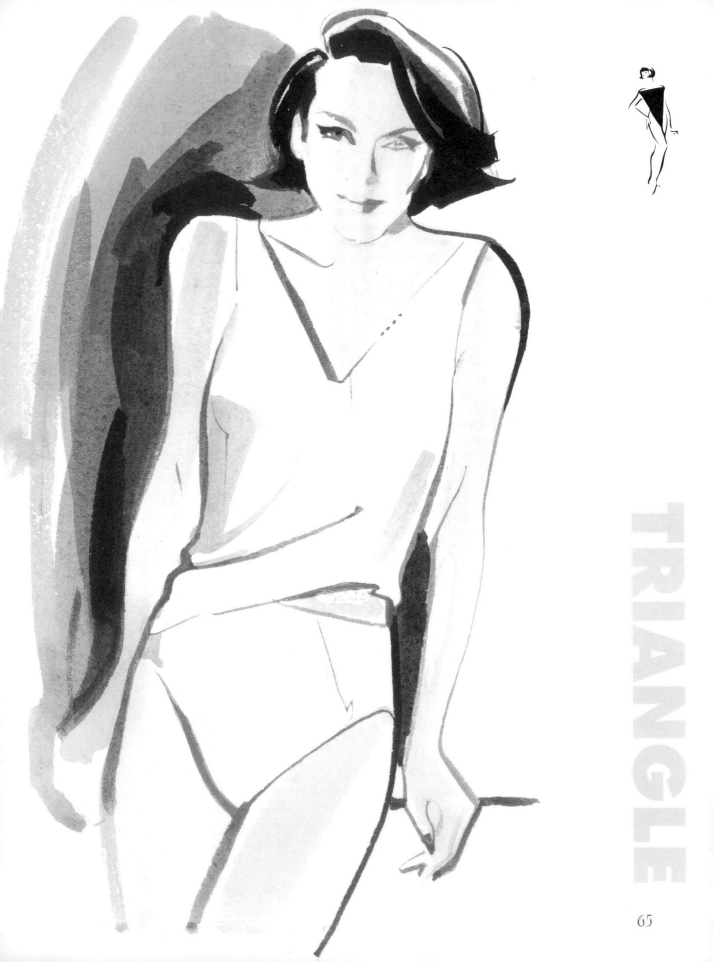

TRIANGLE

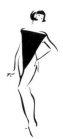

WEEK THREE
Your diet

This week can be a danger week. I found with my volunteer dieters that this was when they could lose heart. Weight loss having been really good in the first two weeks now tends to slow down. Boredom or resentment at not being able to indulge in your favourite high-calorie foods may ambush all your good efforts so far.

From talking to clients and from the evidence of my questionnaire I have found that chocolate cravings can be a real problem for some people, especially pre-menstrually. If you find yourself in the stage of miserable craving I think it is better to find a sensible way of dealing with this and I suggest that you try a low-calorie chocolate drink (most of the leading brands are making one) as a safer substitute than demolishing a box of chocolates. The drink tastes chocolatey, gives you a feeling of fullness and comfort and gets rid of that awful sense of deprivation. But don't go getting addicted to this instead!

Triangle types can be very competitive and successful in masculine professions. Often alcohol is the relaxant they turn to at the end of a hard day. This diet has not allowed alcohol because of the wasted calories and also because it can weaken one's resolve. If you're feeling really deprived, then allow yourself one of your favourite cocktails or measure of spirits, or two glasses of wine. Really enjoy it. Look on it as a treat but decide that that is all you're going to have. This is not the beginning of your total breakdown but a reward for coming so far. A treat like this *once a week* will not do you any harm. Enjoy it. Then get right back on the straight and narrow with the next week's diet.

DAY FIFTEEN
Breakfast
Two eggs, scrambled or any style (OR 100 g (4 oz) kipper fillet grilled OR two pieces back bacon, fat removed, grilled OR half 120 g (4 oz) tin sardines in brine, drained) on one slice of wholemeal toast, low-fat spread from daily allowance, cup tea or coffee.

Lunch
225g (8 oz) white fish, grilled or steamed, two small boiled potatoes, large green salad (from permitted list), low-cal dressing, either commercial brand or home-made (see recipe, page 72), two-fruit salad.

Late-afternoon snack
Two pieces of crispbread spread with 25 g (1 oz) anchovy paste, sandwich spread, vegetable pâté or any low-fat pâté, sliced cucumber on top.

Supper
300 ml (½ pt) any non-creamy packet soup or homemade vegetable soup (see recipe, page 75), one slice of wholemeal bread/toast.

DAY SIXTEEN
Breakfast
Same as above.

Lunch
Spaghetti with broccoli (see recipe, page 74), sliced tomato and onion salad with low-cal dressing (see recipe, page 72), one slice of wholemeal bread, banana split (1 tbsp iced vanilla yogurt instead of ice cream).

Late-afternoon snack
25 g (1 oz) packet savoury popcorn.

Supper
Half avocado, 50 g (2 oz) prawns, green salad, low-cal dressing (see recipe, page 72).

DAY SEVENTEEN
Breakfast
Same as above.

Lunch
175 g Tandoori chicken (see recipe, page 76), selection of vegetables (from permitted list), baked apple cooked with two dried apricots as stuffing, 1 tbsp low-fat natural yogurt.

Late-afternoon snack
Large banana.

Supper
Red cabbage, apple & hazelnut salad (see recipe, page 77).

TRIANGLE

Your exercise programme

By now, your floor exercises should be making a difference to the firmness of your tummy, midriff and inner thighs. Increase the number of repetitions as outlined in the box below.

Are you enjoying your exercise enough? I don't want you to continue with such an energetic regime if you're finding it gruelling and too much like hard labour. Listen to your body and pamper it as well as working out vigorously. How about an aromatherapy massage? Get some ready-mixed massage oil from your chemist and ask a friend or your partner to massage it into your shoulders and back while you relax in a warm quiet room.

Perhaps you might enjoy taking up swimming regularly if you haven't already. It is the perfect exercise if you can keep up a steady stroke for about half an hour. Try it.

EXERCISE REPETITIONS: WEEK THREE	
Modified Cat Stretch	6
Stomach Clincher	8
Inner Thigh Trimmer	4

DAY EIGHTEEN

Breakfast
Same as above, but *not* eggs.

Lunch
Baked potato, 110 g (4 oz) baked beans, two back rashers bacon, trimmed and grilled, low-cal coleslaw or homemade with creamy low-cal dressing (see recipe, page 72).

Late-afternoon snack
50 g (2 oz) olives, raw carrot, celery sticks, 1 tbsp hummus.

Supper
One poached egg on spinach (frozen or fresh, any amount), one wholemeal roll or slice of bread.

DAY NINETEEN

Breakfast
Same as above.

Lunch
Stir-fry beef with mange-tout (see recipe, page 75), green vegetables (from permitted list), boiled or steamed, orange.

Late-afternoon snack
Two crispbreads spread with 25 g (1 oz) fish paste, or low-fat pâté, sliced cucumber on top.

Supper
Baked pepper salad (see recipe, page 77), one wholemeal roll.

DAY TWENTY

Breakfast
Same as above.

Lunch
175 g (6 oz) fresh (grilled) or tinned tuna (in brine not oil), steamed vegetables (from permitted list), 40 g (1½ oz) rice (dried weight, preferably brown) boiled, two-fruit salad.

Late-afternoon snack
Cereal bar (under 100 cals).

Supper
Tabbouleh (see recipe, page 77) in wholemeal pitta bread.

DAY TWENTY-ONE

Breakfast
Same as above.

Lunch
Quarter chicken, roasted/grilled, one wholemeal roll or slice of bread, large mixed salad (from permitted list), low-cal dressing (see recipe, page 72), ginger banana (see recipe, page 79).

Late-afternoon snack
Apple and orange.

Supper
Quick pea soup (see recipe, page 76), one slice of wholemeal bread.

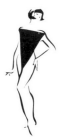

WEEK FOUR
Positive action: start at the top

JUST AS clothes which are angular and chic suit a Triangle-shaped woman best, so do straight and swingy or short and sharp hairstyles. Soft, wavy, romantic hair looks dull and untidy on you—and at odds with your broad-shouldered frame. If you have naturally curly hair, however, it will look much better on you either if you wear it short and spiky, or if you want it longer, in a bob with a straight club cut at the back.

Always remember that it is a geometric feeling which you are aiming for. But do treat yourself to a good cut with a hair stylist who will take into consideration the weight and wave of your own hair and the shape of your face.

If you want to change the colour of your hair, bear in mind that its natural tone is the one which suits your skin and eye colour best. Unless you are aiming for a dramatic look (dark-haired Madonna was never meant to be a blonde), keep within your natural colour range. Dramatic changes can look sensational when you're young (and can afford an expensive professional style—and its maintenance), but they are hardening and ageing to older skins.

Professionally done high- and low-lights can be the most

flattering way of adding zing to your hair without clashing with the rest of your colouring. But it can be expensive. I would always say that if you had to choose, a good cut is the priority. Your own hair colour, glossy and healthy on this diet, will then look as exciting as can be.

TRIANGLE

'I felt very healthy throughout, especially with the exercise. I never felt really hungry, and the extra piece of fruit was a help at about four o'clock.'

Carole

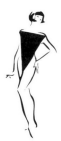

WEEK FOUR
Your diet

You are over the danger period of that third week. Although you may be disappointed that the scales do not register quite as much loss as you hoped I'm sure that by now you are feeling so much better—both slimmer and fitter—that you are quite happy to enter your fourth week. If Week Three had marked a plateau in your weight loss, then by the end of this fourth week I am pretty certain you will find you have lost *more* than you hoped.

DAY TWENTY-TWO
Breakfast
Two eggs, scrambled or any style (OR 100 g (4 oz) kipper fillet grilled OR half 120 g (4 oz) tin sardines in brine) on one slice of wholemeal toast, low-fat spread from daily allowance, cup of tea or coffee.
Lunch
Salade Niçoise (see recipe, page 76), one wholemeal roll, mango, paw paw, or two pieces of fruit from permitted list.
Late-afternoon snack
25 g (1 oz) packet savoury popcorn.
Supper
Ratatouille (see recipe, page 74).

DAY TWENTY-THREE
Breakfast
Same as above.
Lunch
Kyoto Trout Salad (see recipe, page 75), piece of wholemeal bread, low-fat spread from daily allowance, 50 g (2 oz) prunes stewed.
Late-afternoon snack
25 g (1 oz) packet twiglets, OR two crispbreads spread with marmite.
Supper
Green salad with four pecan nuts, low-cal dressing (see recipe, page 72).

DAY TWENTY-FOUR
Breakfast
Same as above, but not eggs.

Lunch
Spanish omelette (see recipe, page 76), one slice of wholemeal bread, large salad (from permitted list), 150 g (5 oz) low-fat fruit yogurt.
Late-afternoon snack
Large banana.
Supper
225 g (8 oz) baked beans on one slice of wholemeal toast.

DAY TWENTY-FIVE
Breakfast
Same as above.
Lunch
Chick pea curry (see recipe, page 74), 50 g (2 oz) rice (dried weight, preferably brown) boiled, steamed broccoli, carrots, or any other vegetables from permitted list, one piece of fruit.
Late-afternoon snack
Cereal bar (under 100 cals).
Supper
Stuffed tomatoes (see recipe, page 73), one piece of crispbread.

DAY TWENTY-SIX
Breakfast
Same as above.
Lunch
Stir-fry chicken and vegetables (see recipe, page 72), 210 g (8 oz) can of any fruit in own juice.
Late-afternoon snack
Two pieces of crispbread spread with 25 g (1 oz) low-fat pâté, sliced cucumber on top.
Supper
Baked pepper and anchovy (see recipe, page 77), one wholemeal roll.

DAY TWENTY-SEVEN
Breakfast
Same as above.
Lunch
200 g (7 oz) white fish (grilled, steamed or baked), broccoli, courgettes, or any other vegetables (from permitted list), one wholemeal roll, stewed prunes

Celebration treat:
buy something RED

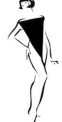

You've got there. Four weeks of a new way of eating and an exercise programme both of which are tailor-made for your body type and I hope you are really feeling more energetic, more attractive, more *you*. To celebrate, I would like to suggest that you go and buy yourself something red. It can be anything from a red scarf or handkerchief to red earrings, a jersey or—if you're feeling really triumphant—a red dress.

But remember, there are many shades of red. There are blue reds and orange reds; clear bright reds or muted, blended reds; light or deep reds. Before buying yourself your red treat hold it under your chin to check it is a flattering red for *you*. The right red will give you a healthy glow, and your skin, hair and eyes will look more vibrant. The wrong red will make you look pale and washed out. Any blemishes and dark shadows on your face are emphasized by the wrong colours.

Red is a marvellous colour. It lifts the spirits. It makes a definite statement; not 'poor 'little over-weight mousy me, please let me pass by, unseen in the crowd', but rather, 'I AM FULL OF LIFE! I AM CONFIDENT, I AM HAPPY, LOOK AT ME!'

---

and apricots (two of each).
Late-afternoon snack
Orange and apple.
Supper
Small baked potato, 1 dessertsp hummus, green side salad.

DAY TWENTY-EIGHT
Breakfast
Same as above.
Lunch
Vegetable casserole (see recipe, page 73), 50 g (2 oz) rice (dried weight, preferably brown) boiled, green salad (from permitted list), low-cal dressing (see recipe, page 72), baked apple with two chopped dates as stuffing, 1tbsp fromage frais (8% fat).
Late-afternoon snack
One slice of wholemeal toast spread with fish paste or low-fat pâte.
Supper
Half avocado, 50 g (2 oz) prawns, green salad (from permitted list), low-cal dressing (see recipe, page 72).

Your exercise programme

The exercise repetitions are outlined in the box below.

You of all the body shapes don't need much encouragement to exercise but I hope that by now you are established in some regular routine of aerobic activity, sports or exercise classes. By now you should really be seeing the benefits in toned-up muscles, extra weight loss and improved circulation and spirits.

There is a 'feel good' factor to exercising which cannot be over-emphasized. If you're doing the exercise that suits your body type and disposition it undoubtedly lifts the spirits, makes you generally more positive about yourself, more in tune with your body—and less likely to neglect and abuse it with junk food.

Here's to a fitter, happier you!

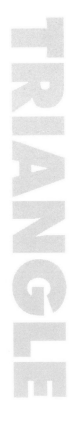

EXERCISE REPETITIONS: WEEK FOUR	
Modified Cat Stretcher	6
Stomach Clincher	8
Inner Thigh Trimmer	4

RECIPE SUPPLEMENT

Low-Cal Dressing

(Make up a jar and use on salads when necessary: 1 dessertsp = 40 calories)

3 tbsp good olive oil
3 tbsp water
3 tbsp wine or cider vinegar
1 clove garlic, crushed
½ tsp salt
1 tsp dried tarragon

1 Put all the ingredients into a screw top jar and shake. Let stand a few hours before using.
2 To vary, use different herbs, or leave out garlic and add 1 tsp capers, liquidise the dressing in a blender. Or add 1 tsp Dijon mustard and 3 tsp apple juice instead of water.

Stir-Fry Chicken and Vegetables

(Serves 1)

25 g (1 oz) brown rice
1 tsp low-fat spread from daily allowance
100 g (4 oz) chicken breast, skinned and sliced
    coarsely
1 Spanish onion, sliced finely
3 sticks celery, sliced
75 g (3 oz) mushrooms, sliced
225 g (8 oz) bean sprouts (fresh or tinned)
2 carrots, coarsely grated
soy sauce/tamari to taste

1 Cook rice in boiling water.
2 In heavy frying pan or wok melt low-fat spread, fry chicken slices until they begin to change colour.
3 Add the prepared vegetables, onion first, then celery, mushrooms, and lastly bean sprouts and carrot.

4 Add splash of soy sauce/tamari to taste. Serve on drained rice.

Creamy Low-Cal Dressing

(Make up a jar and use when necessary: 1 dessertsp = 10 calories)

100 g (4 oz) low-fat cottage cheese
100 g (4 oz) low-fat natural yogurt
½ green pepper, chopped
4 sliced radishes
2 dessertsp chives
1 dessertsp poppy seeds
salt, pepper and pinch basil/oregano to taste

1 Put all ingredients into a blender or food processor. Keep in a jar and use on coleslaw, mixed salads, or in baked potatoes.

Tofu Stir-Fry

(Serves 1)

50 g (2 oz) brown rice
110 g (4 oz) tofu
1 tsp vegetable oil
1 tsp tamari/soy sauce
1 stalk celery, sliced
wedge of white cabbage, coarsely shredded
110 g (4 oz) bean sprouts
25 g (1 oz) water chestnuts (optional)
2 tsp cornflour
1 tsp water
2 tsp tamari/soy sauce

1 Put rice on to boil.
2 Cut tofu into bite-sized pieces.
3 Heat oil in frying pan. Put tofu in pan, sprinkle with tamari/soy sauce. Carefully brown the tofu sides and put aside.

4 Add celery and cabbage to pan, stir-fry 3 minutes. Add bean sprouts and water chestnuts, stir-fry for another 3 minutes.

5 Mix cornflour with water and tamari/soy sauce. Pour mixture over vegetables and stir well. Add tofu, mix gently and cover.

6 Steam for a few minutes until sauce is thickened.

7 Serve with boiled, drained rice.

Cheese-Baked Cauliflower

(Serves 1)

half large head cauliflower
1 egg
1 tbsp skimmed milk
generous pinch dill
25 g (1 oz) cheddar/emmenthal, grated
1 tbsp curd/low-fat soft cheese
salt, pepper

1 Heat oven to 190°C (375°F, gas mark 5)

2 Break cauliflower head into florets, steam or boil in minimum amount of water until just soft.

3 Beat together egg, milk, dill, cheeses, and season.

4 Put cooked cauliflower in small casserole dish, pour on cheesy mixture, cover with lid or foil and cook for about 10 minutes, when egg will have begun to set and cheese to melt.

Stir-Fry Vegetables and Rice

(Serves 1)

50 g (2 oz) brown rice
2 tsp sesame/vegetable oil
1 clove garlic, chopped fine
pinch ginger (1 tsp fresh grated)
selection of vegetables from permitted list (chopped finely, to fill 450 ml [16 fl oz] measuring jug)
25 g (1 oz) cheddar cheese, grated
tamari/soy sauce

1 Put rice on to boil.

2 Heat oil in large frying pan, add garlic and ginger, then add vegetables needing most cooking, ie carrots and any other root vegetables.

3 Stir constantly, adding the vegetables that need less cooking as you go along, ie spring onions, green peppers, mushrooms, bean sprouts. Add a little water if necessary to prevent sticking. Cook until tender/crisp.

4 Serve cooked rice with vegetables, sprinkle cheese on top and add tamari/soy sauce to taste.

Stuffed Tomatoes

(Serves 1)

3 medium sized tomatoes
½ cup cooked rice (brown)
2 pecan nuts, broken
50 g (2 oz) low-fat (curd) cheese
2 tbsp chives/spring onions
pinch dried basil
salt, pepper

1 Cut a 'lid' off the top of each tomato, scoop out and chop pulp.

2 Leave tomato shells upside down on kitchen paper to drain.

3 Add cooked rice, nuts, curd cheese, onion and basil to tomato pulp and beat well. Season to taste.

4 Fill tomatoes with stuffing mixture, replace lids, leave to stand a little before serving.

Vegetable Casserole

(Serves 1)

450 g (1 lb) selection of vegetables from permitted list, eg courgettes, mushrooms, broccoli, carrots, peppers, Brussels sprouts

300 ml (½ pint) water
100 g (4 oz) lentils (dry weight)
1 clove garlic, chopped
1 tsp paprika
salt, pepper
1 vegetable stock cube

1 Chop vegetables, not too small, and put in a small casserole with water, lentils, garlic and paprika. Add salt and pepper and crumbled stock cube and cover with lid.

2 Put in moderate oven—180°C (350°F, gas mark 4)—and cook for about 1 hour, or until tender.

Chick Pea Curry

(Serves 1)

75 g (3 oz) dried chick peas soaked overnight
    (or 215 g [7 oz] tinned)
1 small onion, chopped fine
1–2 cloves garlic, chopped fine
2.5cms (1in) fresh ginger root, grated
1 fresh green chilli, finely chopped (optional)
1–2 tsp curry powder (to taste)
2 large, chopped tomatoes, or 215 g (7 oz) tinned
juice of half lemon
salt, pepper
1 tbsp low-fat natural yogurt

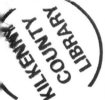

1 If using dried and soaked chick peas, cook in water for an hour or so until tender. Drain cooked or tinned chick peas.
2 In heavy frying pan melt 1 tsp of low-fat margarine from allowance and add onion, garlic, ginger and chilli. Fry gently for 3–4 minutes until soft and browning.
3 Stir in curry powder and cook for another 2 minutes. Add chopped tomatoes and lemon juice.
4 Add chick peas. Stir and simmer 10–15 minutes. Add a little water if curry starts to dry out.
5 Season with salt and pepper, take off heat, stir in yogurt and serve.

Ratatouille

(Serves 1)

225 g (8 oz) courgettes
1 large aubergine
1 green pepper
400 g (15 oz) tin of tomatoes
2 bay leaves
1 large onion, chopped
2 cloves garlic, chopped
salt, pepper

1 Slice the courgettes and aubergine. Core and seed pepper and cut into strips.
2 Place tomatoes in a large saucepan and add the rest of the ingredients.
3 Bring to the boil and simmer for 20 minutes or until vegetables are tender, skim off any sediment. If too much liquid remains, raise heat and boil more vigorously, without the lid, until sauce is thickened.

Seafood Pasta

(Serves 1)

50 g (2 oz) pasta
½ clove garlic, chopped
juice and grated skin ½ lime
75 g (3 oz) prawns
1 tbsp fresh dill (1 tbsp dried)
2 tbsp low-fat natural yogurt
1 tbsp skimmed milk
salt, pepper
2 tsp grated parmesan cheese

1 Cook pasta in boiling water, until tender but *al dente*.
2 Meanwhile put garlic and lime juice and grated skin in small pan and cook gently.
3 When the pasta is nearly ready, add prawns and dill to garlic and lime mixture and heat thoroughly, but don't overcook.
4 Whisk together yogurt and milk and add to the mixture. Heat thoroughly, *but do not boil*. Season to taste.
5 Drain pasta, pour sauce over and sprinkle on parmesan.

Spaghetti with Broccoli

(Serves 1)

1 clove garlic, chopped fine
1 tsp of low-fat spread from daily allowance
175 g (6 oz) broccoli
4–5 tbsp water
50 g (2 oz) spaghetti or other pasta
salt, pepper
2 tsp grated parmesan cheese

1 Gently fry garlic in low-fat spread for 1–2 minutes.
2 Dice broccoli and add to garlic in pan, stir for 2 minutes. Add water, cover and simmer for 10 minutes until broccoli stem is softening. If pan is dry, add a little more water.
3 Cook pasta in pan of lightly salted boiling water for about 7–8 minutes until al dente.
4 Drain pasta and toss with broccoli (which should have a little garlicky juice). Season with salt and milled pepper to taste and sprinkle parmesan on top.

Vegetable Soup

(4 Servings)

1 medium size onion
1 medium size potato
1 medium size parsnip
100 g (4 oz) carrots
25 g (1 oz) low-fat spread from daily allowance
2 tbsp chopped parsley
½ tsp mixed herbs
nutmeg to taste
1.2 l (2 pt) vegetable stock (or 2 cubes)
1 small leek
50 g (2 oz) cabbage
salt, pepper

1 Chop onion, potato, parsnip and carrots. Melt half the low-fat spread in a saucepan and sauté the vegetables gently stirring occasionally, until the onion is transparent.
2 Add parsley, herbs, nutmeg and stock and bring to the boil. Cover and simmer for 30 minutes.
3 Cool a little and then liquidise in blender.
4 Meanwhile, finely shred the leek and cabbage and sauté them in the remaining low-fat spread until just softening. Add to blended soup, simmer gently for 10 minutes. Adjust seasoning.

Kyoto Trout Salad

(Serves 1)

1 medium size trout, skinned and filleted
juice of 2 lemons
1 carrot
5-cm (2-in) piece of cucumber
handful of lambs' tongue lettuce (or rocket/frisée)
¼ avocado, sliced
¼ red pepper, cut in strips
¼ green pepper, cut in strips
1 tsp olive oil

1 Put trout fillets into a shallow bowl and pour over lemon juice. Leave all day, or overnight to marinade, turning occasionally.
2 Drain fillets from lemon juice and cut into chunks.
3 Cut carrot and cucumber lengthwise, into fine sticks, and mix with the lambs' tongue lettuce, avocado slices and red and green pepper. Add the trout pieces.
4 Arrange on your plate and trickle the olive oil over the mixture.

Bean and Lentil Salad

(Serves 1)

75 g (3 oz) (cooked weight) cooked or tinned kidney beans
25 g (1 oz) (cooked weight) green lentils
¼ red pepper, cut in strips
¼ green pepper, cut in strips
¼ spanish onion, cut in fine rings
1 tsp lemon juice
1 tsp olive oil
salt, pepper
handful of chopped parsley and/or chives

1 Put the beans, lentils, peppers and onion rings in a bowl.
2 Pour on the lemon juice and the oil and mix well. Season and toss the parsley and or chives on top.

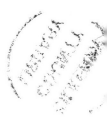

Stir-Fry Beef with Mange-Tout

(Serves 1)

75 g (3 oz) beef fillet, cut across grain into thin strips
soy sauce
1 tsp vegetable (or sesame) oil
75 g (3 oz) mange-tout, topped and tailed
dash of sherry

1 Sprinkle beef strips with soy sauce and leave for at least an hour.
2 Preheat wok or heavy frying pan with 1 tsp oil.
3 Stir-fry beef strips for 2 minutes. Add prepared mange-tout and continue to stir.
4 After another 2 minutes, or when cooked, pour in a teaspoon of soy sauce and a dash of sherry. Mix all ingredients together for another minute and serve.

Tandoori Chicken

(Serves 1)

1 tsp Tandoori Masala barbecue powder
1 clove garlic, minced or crushed
1 dessertsp tomato purée
1 tbsp natural low-fat yogurt
¼ chicken portion

1 Mix all the spices and tomato purée into yogurt.
2 Cut long slices in the chicken flesh and cover with the yogurt mixture, working it into the flesh. Leave for as long as possible, preferably all day or overnight.
3 Scrape off any excess mixture and grill for 15 minutes each side, or until properly cooked (stick a skewer into the thickest part and make sure the juices are no longer pink).

Quick Pea Soup

(Serves 1)

100 g (4 oz) frozen peas
300 ml (½ pt) chicken OR vegetable stock (or ½ cube)
½–1 tbsp fresh mint (optional)
1 tbsp fromage frais 8% OR natural yogurt
salt, pepper

1 Simmer peas in stock for 2–3 minutes, or until cooked. Add chopped mint, if using.
2 Liquidize the soup with the fromage frais or yogurt.
3 Re-heat gently if you need to, but *do not boil*. Season to taste.

Mushroom Omelette

(Serves 1)

1 tsp low-fat spread from daily allowance
100 g (4 oz) sliced mushrooms
2 eggs
1 tbsp fromage frais 8% OR natural yogurt
salt, pepper
fresh parsley or other herbs

1 In small heavy frying pan melt the low-fat spread and add the mushrooms.
2 Cook gently until browning. Remove from pan.

3 Beat eggs with fromage frais or yogurt, add seasoning and pour mixture into pan.
4 With wooden spoon, draw in the setting edges towards the centre. When set, but still quite moist, arrange mushrooms and parsley on one half of pan and fold other half of omelette over.
5 Serve on warm plate.

Spanish Omelette

(Serves 1)

1 tsp low-fat spread from daily allowance
100 g (4 oz) prepared vegetables, eg sliced courgettes, red pepper, mushrooms, peas, fine chopped carrot
1 dessertsp chopped parsley
salt, pepper
2 eggs

1 Heat the fat in a small heavy-bottomed frying pan.
2 Add the mixed vegetables and stir until they begin to soften, turn heat low and cook until *al dente*, stirring frequently.
3 Add chopped parsley, salt and pepper.
4 Lightly beat eggs, season lightly and pour mixture onto vegetables in pan.
5 Stir gently with a fork until eggs begin to set. Serve from pan.

Salade Niçoise

(Serves 1)

lettuce leaves
100 g (4 oz) cooked green beans, cooled
2 tomatoes, sliced
100 g (4 oz) tuna in brine
1 hard boiled egg, quartered
4 anchovy fillets, drained
4 black olives
1 dessertsp low-cal dressing (see page 72)
salt, pepper

1 Arrange a bed of lettuce leaves, add the beans and sliced tomatoes.
2 Pile the drained and flaked tuna in the middle and arrange the egg quarters around the edge.
3 Garnish with the anchovies and black olives. Sprinkle on the dressing and season to taste.

Red Cabbage, Apple and Hazelnut Salad

(Serves 1)

175 g (6 oz) red cabbage
1 eating apple (cox/russet)
25 g (1 oz) raisins
1 dessertsp low-cal dressing (see page 72)
25 g (1 oz) hazelnuts

1 Wash and shred cabbage finely. Core and chop apple coarsely.
2 Combine cabbage, apple and raisins in a bowl, pour on dressing and mix well. Ideally leave for about 2 hours before eating.
3 Sprinkle on chopped hazelnuts just before serving.

Tabbouleh

(Serves 1)

This dish traditionally comes loaded with olive oil but this is a recipe for a much less oil-rich (and therefore less calorie-rich) version.

40 g (1½ oz) bulgar/cracked wheat
4–6 spring onions, finely chopped
2 tbsp fresh parsley, finely chopped
1 tbsp fresh mint
7.5-cms (3-in) piece of cucumber
1–2 tomatoes, chopped
juice of ½ lemon
1 dessertsp low-cal dressing (see above)
salt, pepper

1 Pour boiling water over the wheat and leave for 10 minutes to swell. Drain in a sieve and with your hands squeeze out as much excess water as possible.
2 Put wheat in a bowl and add chopped onions, parsley, mint, cucumber and tomatoes (minus their seeds and watery pulp).
3 Mix in lemon juice, low-cal dressing, salt and pepper to taste.
4 If possible, allow to stand for a while to let flavours blend.

Baked Pepper Salad

(Serves 1)

2 red firm fresh peppers
1 dessertsp low-cal dressing (see above)
fresh parsley (optional)

1 Heat up grill. Place whole red pepper under grill and cook each side until the flesh is charred and blistering.
2 When all sides have blistered and peppers have cooled enough to touch, run under cold water and peel off outer, burnt skin.
3 Slice in half, de-seed and de-core, and slice flesh lengthways into strips.
4 Place on side-plate and dribble low-cal dressing over strips. Serve with chopped fresh parsley if available.

Baked Pepper & Anchovy

(Serves 1)

1 fresh red pepper
2 anchovy fillets, drained
2 cloves garlic, sliced fine
1 tomato sliced into four
1tsp good olive oil

1 Set oven to moderately high 190°C (375°F, gas mark 5).
2 Quarter red pepper, de-core and de-seed, and place skin side down in small ovenproof dish.
3 In each quarter place half anchovy fillet, 3 slices of garlic and slice of tomato.
4 Brush each quarter with olive oil.
5 Cook in oven for 30–40 minutes. Serve hot or cold.

Crudités with Crab Dip

(Serves 2)

175 g (6 oz) can of crabmeat
150 g (5 oz) low-fat natural yogurt
1 tsp lemon juice
salt, pepper
2 carrots
1.3 cm (½ in) cucumber
2 sticks of celery
1 red/green pepper

1 Drain brine off crabmeat and mix with yogurt and lemon juice. Season with salt and pepper to taste.
2 Wash and slice carrots, cucumber and celery into strips.
3 Halve red/green pepper, de-seed and cut into strips.
4 Put crab dip into a small bowl and arrange vegetables on a plate.

Mushroom and Pepper Risotto

(Serves 1)

1 clove garlic, minced or finely chopped
½ medium onion, chopped
1 tsp olive oil
175 g (6 oz) mushrooms (ideally large, field
   mushrooms), diced
½ green/red pepper, de-seeded and diced
50 g (2 oz) white round grain rice (preferably risotto
   rice, but pudding rice will do)
1 vegetable stock cube
1 dessertsp sherry (optional)
handful of parsley, chopped
4 spring onions, chopped (optional)

1 Gently fry the garlic and onion in oil in a heavy, medium-sized frying pan, until transparent.
2 Add mushrooms and diced pepper and stir for a minute or so, then add rice and continue stirring.
3 Make 300 ml (½ pt) of vegetable stock with cube and add this to the rice and vegetable mixture. Add sherry, if using it.
4 Simmer gently in the uncovered pan for 25–30 minutes until the rice is cooked. If the mixture dries out before the rice is properly cooked, add a little

more water.
5 Sprinkle the parsley and optional spring onions on top and serve.

Fish Florentine

(Serves 1)

175 g (6 oz) fillet of white fish
120 g (4 oz) frozen chopped spinach, thawed
25 g (1 oz) parmesan or cheddar cheese, grated
pepper

1 Place fillet in bottom of small, shallow baking dish.
2 Having squeezed all excess moisture out of the spinach, place over fish.
3 Sprinkle with cheese and season with pepper.
4 Bake in hot oven, 200°C (400°F, gas mark 6) for 20 minutes.

Crunchy Chicken Salad

(Serves 1)

1 chicken breast
1 carrot, diced
1 tbsp low-fat natural yogurt
1 tsp calorie-reduced mayonnaise
1 small clove garlic, chopped small
pinch paprika
salt, pepper
4 spring onions, sliced
½ eating apple, cored and cubed
½ bunch watercress, minus stalks
2 tbsp shredded red or hard white cabbage
½ red pepper, de-seeded and sliced

1 Put chicken breast in small pan, cover with water and simmer for 25 minutes, remove skin and add carrots. Cook for another 5 minutes, until chicken is cooked and carrots still firm..
2 Drain and cool. Cut chicken flesh into strips.
3 Mix yogurt and mayonnaise and add garlic, paprika, salt and pepper to taste.
4 Mix chicken strips with carrots, spring onions, apple, watercress leaves, hard cabbage, red pepper. Add dressing mixture. Toss and chill in fridge before serving.

Papaya and Mango Fruit Salad

(Serves 2)

1 ripe papaya
1 ripe mango
rind and juice of ½ lime

1 Peel, halve and de-seed papaya, slice lengthwise and then cut into cubes.
2 Peel mango and slice flesh off stone, cut into cubes.
4 Mix fruit together in a bowl with finely grated zest and juice of half a lime.
5 Divide into two servings.

Orange Sorbet

(Serves 1)

1 dessertsp lemon juice
1 tsp liquid honey
grated rind of ½ orange
half 175 g (8 oz) can unsweetened orange juice
1 small egg white
slices of orange to garnish

1 Mix lemon juice with honey and make it up to 150 ml (¼ pint) with warm water.
2 Add orange rind and juice and pour mixture into a 600 ml (1 pint) bowl and put in freezer.
3 When half frozen, mash with a fork into a semi-frozen pulp.
4 Whisk egg white until stiff and fold into the mixture with a metal spoon.
5 Return to freezer and freeze until firm.
6 Before serving, leave it in the refrigerator for 15–20 minutes to soften it slightly. Serve with an orange twist.

Rhubarb Fool

(Serves 1)

175 g (6 oz) rhubarb
1 lemon
liquid sweetener
150 g (5 oz) low-fat natural yogurt

1 Top and tail the rhubarb, then wash and cut into chunks.
2 Put rhubarb into a small saucepan with 1 tbsp lemon juice, ½ tsp lemon zest and 1 tbsp water. Simmer gently.
3 When cooked, add liquid sweetener to taste.
4 Put aside to cool. Then blend mixture in a liquidizer.
5 Pour rhubarb into a bowl and fold in the yogurt. Chill and serve.

Ginger Bananas

(Serves 1)

1 ripe banana
1 piece of crystallized ginger, chopped
few almond flakes
1 tbsp fromage frais 8%/frozen yogurt

1 Slice banana into pudding bowl.
2 Sprinkle ginger over bananas, top with almonds and serve with fromage frais or frozen yogurt.